BETTER SEX IN NO TIME

AN ILLUSTRATED GUIDE
FOR BUSY COUPLES

JOSEY VOGELS
FOREWORD BY JENNY BLOCK

CLEiS
PRESS

Published in the United States by Cleis Press, Inc.,
2246 Sixth Street, Berkeley, California 94710.

Printed in South Korea.
Cover design: Scott Idleman/Blink
Cover photograph: B2M Productions/Getty Images
Text design: Collins
Illustrations: Kveta/Three in a Box

First Edition.
10 9 8 7 6 5 4 3 2 1

Trade paper ISBN: 978-1-62778-071-1
E-book ISBN: 978-1-62778-083-4

Better Sex in No Time was originally published in Canada by Collins, an imprint of HarperCollins Publishers Ltd.

Part 4 was first published by Collins, an imprint of HarperCollins Publishers Ltd., in 2012, in e-book form only, under the title *50 Degrees Hotter in No Time.*

The author gratefully acknowledges Good for Her in Toronto (goodforher.com) for generously providing the toys that appear in the appendix.

TO DANIEL
for making time

CONTENTS

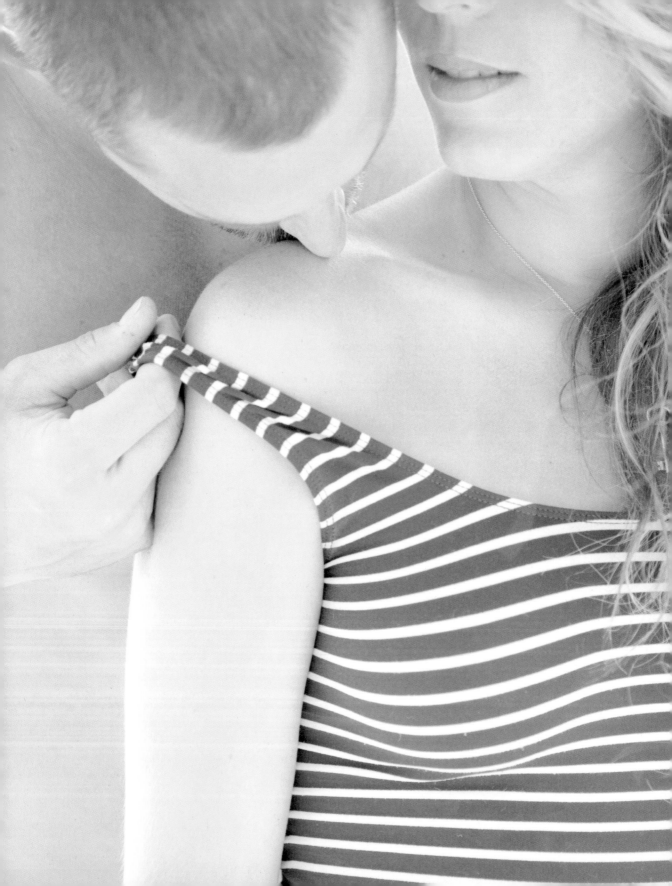

FOREWORD

While you may not actually be able to *make* time, this book will help you discover the loophole—there is time for everything that is important to you. The only question is—what is truly important?

If you're like me, love and sex are very high on your list. So you make sure there is time, because your very existence depends on it. Sadly, we don't always do that, perhaps feeling like sex shouldn't be (or doesn't need to be) a priority in our lives. . . but it has to be.

It's an ugly analogy, but if you had cancer, you would make time for treatment. If you had a loved one who was dying, you would make time for their care. A dearth of love and sex may not seem life threatening. But to a relationship, they are.

A furtive glance across the table. A text that only the two of you will understand. A hand sweeping firmly across your collarbone. These are the kinds of gestures that we have forgotten about and the very same gestures that can open us and breathe new life into our romantic and sexual relationships.

It's no wonder our relationships and deep connections have gone awry. The world is simply too much with us these days. It's near impossible to think about love and romance—let alone sex—when the project is late, the chicken is burnt and the house is wrecked. But if we let the mundane rob us of the sublime, we are lost.

The prospect of this may seem daunting. Perhaps you are in a relatively new partnership, and this seems like too much too soon. How could you do these things with someone you are just starting out with? Or maybe you are in a long-term relationship and this seems almost laughable. How could you do these things with someone who knows you cry at sappy commercials and wear your lucky boxers with Snoopy on them when you get nervous?

That's the glory of this book—it meets you wherever you are and offers you bits, bites and portions that you can do right now. Literally. This minute. From seduction to spice and everything in between. From five seconds to an hour, to all night long. From the perfectly innocent to the deliciously deviant.

It's not rocket science. It's sex. It's romance. It's love. It's playing and teasing and reveling. It's pleasure, and you have a right and a responsibility to it. And your partner does, too. We have to commit to it as we commit to every other part of our well-being. It is no less vital. No less life affirming. No less sacred.

If it were in my power to change the Declaration of Independence, I would rewrite our forefathers' words to include *pleasure* on that list of inherent and inalienable rights.

We are so wholly obsessed with sex, and yet we don't take it seriously. Not really. We let it slip and ebb, and we suffer for it.

You can make time. You *have* to, in fact. And this book will guide you as you do just that on your journey to discovering better sex in no time.

Jenny Block
Author of *Open* and *O Wow!*

IT'S ABOUT TIME

You don't have enough time for sex. I get it. After a busy, stressful day of work, kids, meals, soccer practice, homework and identifying the source of the weird smell coming out of the fridge, it's unrealistic to think you're going to fall into bed and suddenly want to make mad, passionate love. After all, you know you have to get up in a few hours and do it all over again (the work and kids stuff, that is, not the mad, passionate love stuff). Sleep feels like a luxury, so sex feels like something between a fond memory and a chore. But what if instead of being an afterthought — something you'll get to eventually once the rest of life gets out of the way or a task you're just too damn tired for — sex became something you went out of your way to make time for, something you *got excited about,* something that was a reward rather than another item you never seem to get to on your to-do list? Wouldn't that be wonderful?

Stop for a second (you've got at least one free second, don't you?) and think about other things in your life that you go out of your way to make time for. Things you eagerly anticipate, that make you feel relaxed and calm, and that you're never too tired for. What about something like a pedicure? A lovely indulgence, no? Pedicures make you feel pampered, cared for and relaxed. Because you know this, you make time for them, schedule them and look forward to them. Are you ever too tired for a pedicure? Granted, sex can require a little more exertion than a pedicure, but do you see what I mean? The end result makes up for any prep work. And you, big guy, you may not like to relax with a nice facial or back waxing, but maybe you love to get out on the squash court once or twice a week. So you carve time out of your week by scheduling it. You make sure you have all the gear you need. You look forward to it. Squash requires a lot more energy then sex, but you're never too tired for it, are you? In fact, after a good, sweaty game of squash you probably feel more energized, relaxed and good about yourself, right?

In other words, no matter how busy or tired you are, you make time for the things you really *want* to do.

Remember when you were first dating? You *wanted* to have sex all the time. And you constantly wooed each other to get it. You planned dates. You did special things for each other. You made each other feel desirable, admired and cherished all the time because you *wanted* to have sex. You wanted to have sex all the time because it made you feel desirable, admired and cherished. See how that works? Pretty neat, huh? You want to have sex with your partner, so you put effort into making her feel sexy and, lo and behold, she wants to have sex with you, and then because she wants to *keep* having sex with you because you make her feel so sexy, she puts effort into making you feel sexy, which makes you want to keep having sex with her. It all kind of makes you feel sexy, doesn't it?

Sadly, once you've both been satisfactorily snagged and settle into your relationship, the wooing tends to slow down if not stop completely. And, not surprisingly, without the wooing, the desire for sex slows down too.

If you want to find the time for sex, you have to make sex something you both look forward to and are excited about, like pedicures or squash. Once you create the want, you'll be surprised how motivated you are to find the time for sex. Sex will change from something you never seem to get to (not sexy) to something you really look forward to and make time for (very sexy).

So let's return to your original claim: You don't have time for sex. Now, I'd like you to take another second or two (c'mon, I know you're busy, but you can take a couple more seconds) and rephrase that sentence: You aren't making the time for sex because, perhaps, if you were honest with yourself, you've lost the *want* or (if you're craving sexier language) the *desire* for sex that came so easily early in the relationship.

But here's the good news: Creating desire doesn't take as much time as you might think, just a little conscious daily effort. It's like that old saying: How do you eat an elephant? One bite at a time. How do you create want and desire? One sexy thought, one kind gesture, one passionate kiss, one hot date at a time.

Let me use another analogy. Say you want to lose ten pounds. You carry that goal around with you every day but you can't seem to find the motivation to do anything about it. One day you decide to walk instead of taking the bus. You feel good. You feel motivated. The next day, you pack a few healthier snacks. You forgo the chips while watching TV. One morning, you notice your pants are a little looser. Woohoo! This motivates you even more. You take things up a notch by adding a little jogging or using a set of weights every night. Finally, one morning, you step on the scale and you're ten pounds lighter. Instead of being overwhelmed and ultimately defeated by focusing on the end goal, you started by doing little things every day. The more success you had, the more motivated you became, which helped you make more of an effort by adding new challenges. The next thing you knew, you were having more sex, I mean, you'd lost the ten pounds. And it just took a little bit of time every day.

Like wanting to lose ten pounds, "finding more time for sex" is a vague and overwhelming goal. What do you mean by "sex" anyway? If you suddenly do find yourselves with a two-hour or even a ten-minute chunk of time for sex, it's going to be hard to suddenly flip on the "sex" switch if there hasn't been any buildup of desire. So let's start by focusing on simple ways to create desire in each other, the baby steps (or elephant bites if you like) that will motivate you and get you back on track to wanting, and ultimately finding time for, sex, be it a quickie, a longie or all the wonderful things in between.

"But I don't want sex to feel like losing ten pounds," you say, balking. "That's not hot. Besides, when we first dated, we didn't have to put any effort into desire. It just happened. We couldn't keep our hands off each other. And sex was always spontaneous. We'd be groping in the cab on the way home from the restaurant and barely in the door before we were naked and doing it on the hallway floor."

Right. Can I let you in on a wee secret? All that sex you had in the beginning may have been super-hot but it wasn't truly spontaneous. No, really. Think about it. You had each other in a constantly heightened state. You flirted endlessly. Each kiss was full of meaning and intensity. Every time you got naked, it felt as if you were seeing the other person's body for the first time. When you were apart, you were thinking about the last time you were together and anticipating the next time, probably planning what you'd wear, what you'd say, where you'd have sex and what new things you might try. And when you finally reconnected, you "spontaneously" couldn't keep your hands off each other. Well, duh. You may not have felt like you were working at seduction and creating anticipation, buildup and, ultimately, desire, but you were. All the time. It just didn't feel like work. After you've been coupled for a while, you start to spend more time thinking about the fact that he didn't pick his socks up off the very hallway floor where you were having sex in the early days. Or that she's wearing the same comfy sweats she wore in front of the TV last night. All of which pretty much dulls desire if not kills it.

The more romance you create and the more you seduce one another in small ways every day, the less it will feel like work. You'll reignite the anticipation, excitement and longing you once felt. Sex will start to feel spontaneous again because you both really want it. And you'll miraculously find time for sex because it's easy to make time for something you both really want to do. It's that simple.

I'm going to give you lots of ideas to jump-start desire and get your sex life back on track, whether you have five minutes or five hours. Some suggestions may feel awkward at first, especially if your sex life feels a bit rusty. But eventually not only will sex feel natural again, the positive results will motivate you to take things up a notch. Just start by promising to devote five minutes a day to connecting sexually with your partner, and it will have a ripple effect. It's like getting out for a short run. Once you get in the habit and realize how good it feels, you'll want to devote more time to it. Before you know it, you and your partner will be motivated to devote entire evenings or even a whole weekend to sex. It will become something you eagerly seek out rather than another chore on your to-do list.

With this book and a little effort, you'll be having better sex . . . in no time.

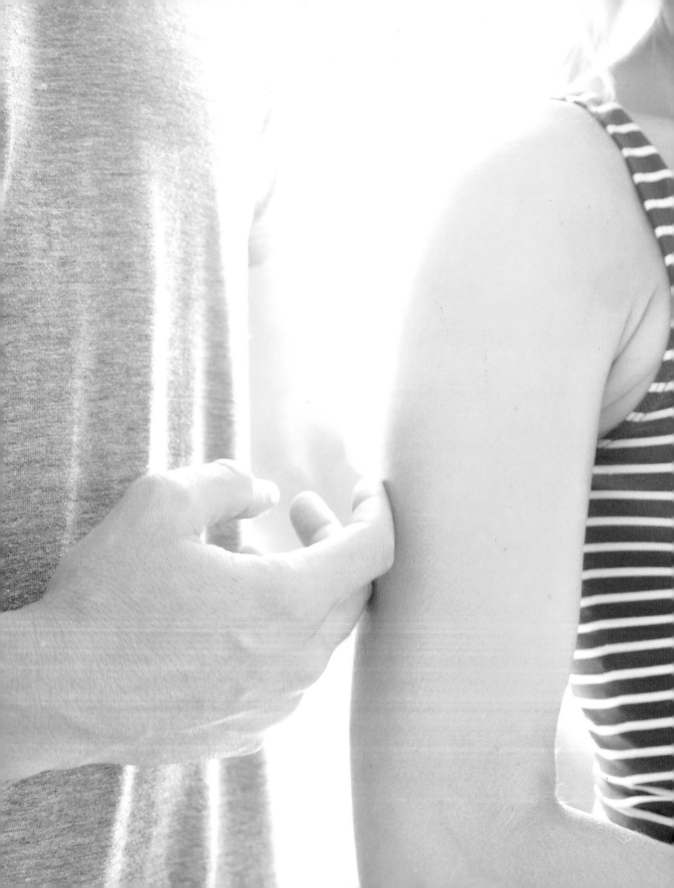

1

SEDUCTION

Seduction doesn't always have to be a prelude to sex, but it absolutely does have to be an ongoing aspect of your relationship if you want to keep desire and sexual interest alive. It's what makes your partner feel cherished, noticed, pampered, indulged and sexy, even when you're nowhere near the bedroom. If you think seduction is a waste of time, think about this: Spending a bit of time seducing each other on a daily basis actually saves time in the long run because you'll constantly be fired up about each other. When you're constantly fired up, sex won't feel so far out of reach when you do have more time to take things further.

Don't be intimidated. You don't have to be Casanova or Mata Hari to seduce your partner. You can incorporate seduction into your daily routine in simple ways that require no swashbuckling or exotic Indian dancing (but hey, feel free to go for it). Create more romance. Pay attention to the little things. Date. Flirt. Take a few extra seconds to put some meaning and intensity back into your kisses. When you realize the immediate positive effect of these small gestures, you'll wonder why the heck you ever let this aspect of your relationship wane. If daily seduction has never been a big part of your relationship, I guarantee that, if you make the effort, you'll unearth a whole new level of intimacy.

Here I'll show you easy ways to bring more romance into your day-to-day life, and how to flirt with each other so you can rekindle the desire that burned early on in your relationship. I'll tell you how to put some sizzle back into your smooches and how to find the time to date again, along with some ideas for what to do on all those great dates you'll be having. Finally, I bare all—well, technically, you'll bare all—about getting naked in ways that will turn the simple act of taking your clothes off into the act of "do me now, baby!"

Time Challenge

If you have five seconds . . .
While she's making dinner, walk up behind her. Brush your hands along the small of her back, lightly kiss the nape of her neck and walk away.

If you have five minutes . . .
Make a list of all the things he did today that you appreciated and leave it on his pillow.

If you have twenty minutes . . .
Go for a walk together after dinner and reminisce about one of your most memorable early dates. Stop and smooch along the way.

If you have an hour . . .
Write an old-fashioned love letter . . . with a slightly naughty twist. If you're at a loss for words, find a flirty passage from a book that expresses how you feel.

If you have three hours . . .
Hire a professional photographer and do a naked photo shoot together.

If you have all night . . .
Make her favourite dinner and make out on the couch (above the belt only) for dessert.

START WITH THE BASICS

Be genuine.

If your actions feel more dutiful than heartfelt, they will be a turnoff.

Make it personal.

The more significant and meaningful, the better.

Don't equate elaborate with better.

Paying attention to details often has more impact than grandiose displays of affection.

Do it without sex as the goal.

You don't want to imply "I'm only doing this so you'll have sex with me."

Be playful.

Don't take it all too seriously. Relax and have fun.

Be confident.

Being sure of yourself is always sexy.

Don't worry about getting it "right."

A little awkwardness and some fumbling are real, funny and sexy.

Get out of your comfort zone.

They may feel out of character, but unexpected gestures will be appreciated that much more.

Switch it up.

Just because you discover something pushes the right button, don't be afraid to try another button. Variety is, after all, the spice of your sex life.

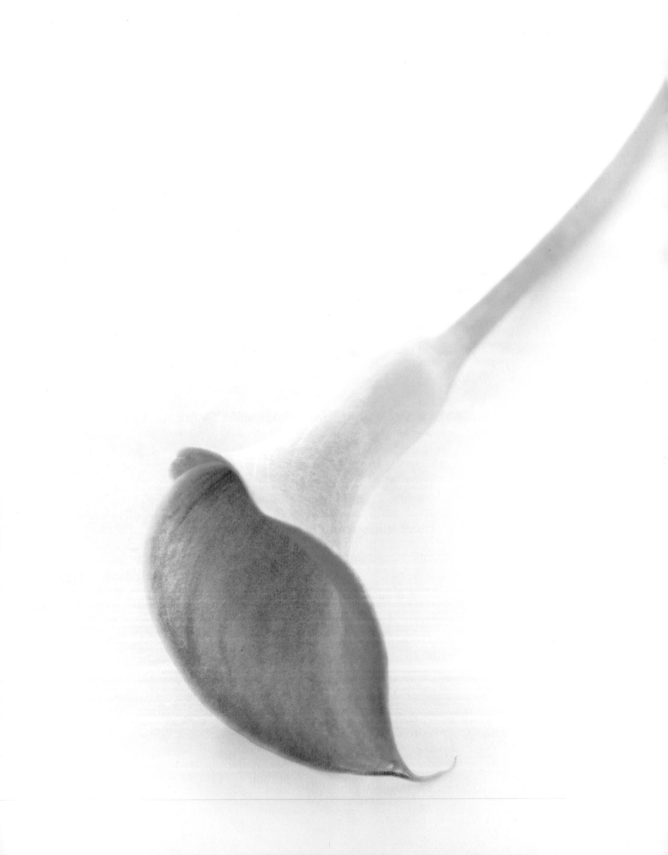

Chapter One
ROMANCE

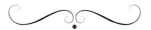

Don't worry, gentlemen, I'm not about to suggest you go out and buy yourself a lute and some tights so you can serenade her under a full moon. I understand that traditional ideas of romance can feel silly and forced if you're not "that" kind of guy. Being romantic doesn't have to mean rose petals on the bed, candlelight and poetry. Those things are romantic, yes, but they are clichéd stereotypes of romance. You can also be romantic simply by doing things that let her know you are paying attention—that you cherish her and want her to feel special and loved. That you "get" her.

Gestures don't have to be elaborate or time-consuming. They just have to say "I'm thinking of you." In fact, why not send her a text right now that says "Just thinking of you." Go. Do it. Done?

Great. That was romantic and it took, what, ten seconds? See, you do have the time to be romantic. It can be as simple as showing your appreciation by complimenting her on handling a tough situation at work or by letting her stay in bed and read the paper while you watch the kids. These things take almost no time but will mean a lot more than you might think.

In fact, whatever the romantic overture, making it meaningful—to her—is the key. You may think that going out and spending lots of money on an elaborate resort getaway will thrill her, but if she's stressed at work, can't possibly take off for a week and hates resorts, she'll feel more resentful that you aren't paying attention and don't understand her. Simply noticing how stressed she is and taking the kids out so she can have an evening to herself is a less grandiose gesture, but it may be more appreciated.

Oh, and ladies? Just because our culture perpetuates the idea that women love romance and men must do the romancing, you're not off the hook, my dears. Your guy also likes to be romanced. He might not put it in quite the same words, but trust me, he wants to feel pampered, cherished, appreciated and special, just as much as you do. He wants to feel that you notice him and are paying attention—that you really "get" him and appreciate him for exactly who he is.

He loves it when you laugh out loud at his goofy jokes while you're out with friends or you tell him that you love his unique ability to make the kids squeal with delight when he plays with them. Things like this remind him why the two of you are so fantastic together. They make him feel close, connected and, bonus for you, more inclined to do lots more special things for you (not that reciprocation is the goal here).

The bottom line is that if you want to create more desire in your relationship, romancing one another is an absolutely necessary building block. Take ten seconds, twenty seconds, even a whole minute out of your day to do something romantic for your partner, and you'll notice a remarkable change: You'll feel more loving toward each other, and the positive feedback will make you want to keep it up, which in turn will make you feel more intimate, open, romantic and, ultimately, sexual toward each other.

TIME to PLAY

Five Minutes or Less
Make a Note of It

Leave a sticky note on the bathroom mirror describing one thing you love about your partner that you'll be thinking about today. Point out how much you adore waking up to her beautiful face every morning or how much you love his sexy lower back.

What's So Funny?

Make each other laugh out loud. Yes, making each other laugh is romantic. Laughter opens and softens hearts. Too often, when relationships become entrenched in the day-to-day, you forget to make each other laugh. Gently teasing (as in playful, nice teasing, not mean-brother type of teasing) one another and interacting like you're new lovers can help remind you. I know a woman whose husband comes charging into the room completely naked, pounces on her and yells "NAKED MAN!" while she's quietly reading a book or watching TV. So romantic, hey? Okay, not every woman will appreciate a naked pounce. The point it, this is something specific between them that he knows cracks her up. It's a unique (albeit kind of weird) little inside joke they share that puts them in that wonderfully romantic "it's just us, baby" bubble. Be it an inside joke or a cheesy pet name, go make your partner dissolve into fits of laughter, right now.

Don't Do It

It's Saturday morning, your day to get things done: the laundry, the grocery shopping and the cleaning. Instead of jumping out of bed and getting right to it, forget the to-do list for five minutes, stay in bed with him and relax as you snuggle and chat about anything other than the day's itinerary. And you, mister? Return the favour by getting up with her to help plow through the chores so you can enjoy free time together later that day.

> 66 If you want to create more desire in your relationship, romancing one another is an absolutely necessary building block. 99

One Hour or Less

You're Soaking in It

When she gets home from work, have a glass of wine poured and a bath running for her. Hand her the glass and tell her to go relax while you prepare dinner. If she's not

---

Quick Tip: Makin' a List

Each of you write down ten romantic things you'd enjoy. Exchange lists and tuck them away. When you're strapped for time and want to do something romantic for your partner, simply consult their list. Yes, it's still romantic even if they came up with the idea. The romance lies in you actually following through and doing it for them.

a bath person, think about what she does to relax, then, whatever it is, set it up so that it's waiting for her to enjoy at the end of a long day.

A Clean Break
If your partner does most of the housework, surprise them by cleaning the bathroom/kitchen/children . . . without being asked (yes, toilet scrubbing can be romantic).

Smooth Move
If he's had a rough day, sit him down, fix him a drink and rub his shoulders. Ask him if he wants to talk about it. If he doesn't, let him simply relax and unwind while you do your magic. If he does, sympathize with him while he vents.

All Night
Movie Night
Make a note of that old movie she mentioned she loves. Buy it for her birthday (or better yet, for no reason at all) and watch it together in bed with a bottle of champagne.

A Lesson in Giving
She says in passing that she's always wanted to learn to salsa dance (or insert whatever it is she's mentioned she'd like to try). You'd rather eat paint. But, knowing how happy it would make her, surprise her with lessons . . . and agree to go with her.

Develop Appreciation
Designate one day a month as "Appreciation Day." That day, each of you carries a note pad around to jot down all the nice things you notice about your partner—physical things about them, sweet things they do, quirky habits you find endearing, funny things they say. That night, over a glass of wine, read the lists out loud to each other.

Game On
Watch the game with him, even (especially) if you're not into that particular sport. Ask questions (maybe during the commercials so you don't interrupt a really important play). He'll love that you're taking an interest, and you'll enjoy the pride he takes in being able to share his knowledge of the game.

> 66 Designate one day a month as 'Appreciation Day.' That day, each of you carries a note pad around to jot down all the nice things you notice about your partner. 99

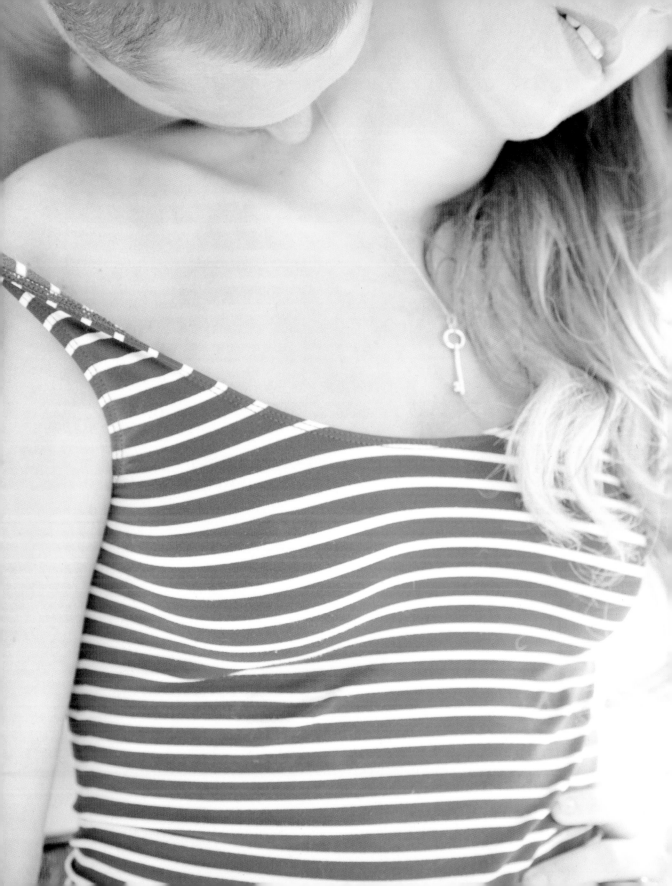

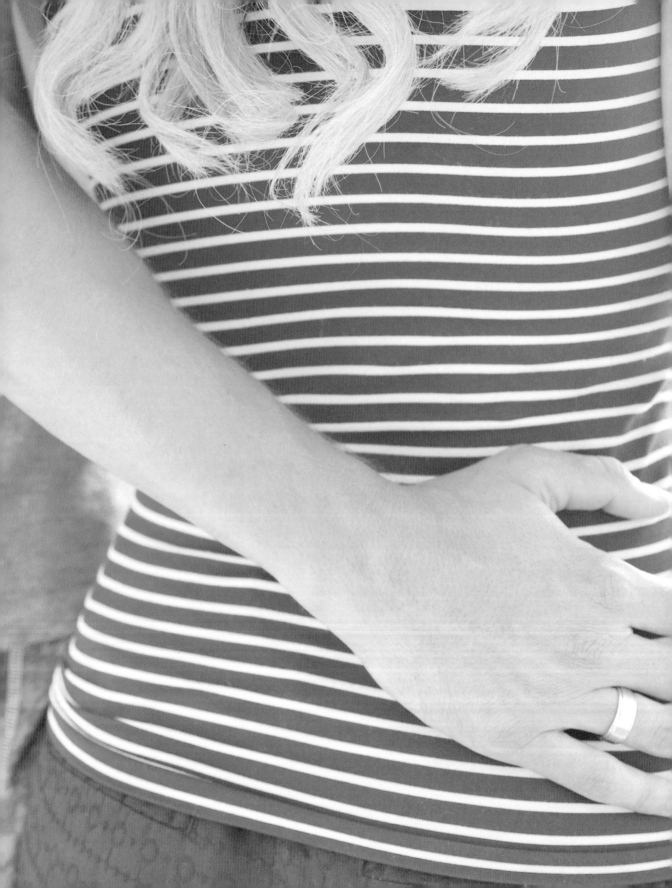

Chapter Two
FLIRT

Flirting is romance's naughty cousin. Where romance is about indulging your partner, flirting is about leaving them wanting more. That's why it's such a great seduction tactic. It's like foreplay's foreplay. Flirting has an edge of naughtiness with a dash of "Oh, goodness, did I really say that?" that gets the juices flowing without anyone having to get naked. Flirting keeps sex on the table (though, just so you know, if you're having sex on the table you're well beyond flirting), even if you don't have time to sit down for a full meal.

You no doubt flirted all the time when you were first dating — when you were working for it (but didn't know you were working). Often, once you're secure in your relationship, you abandon this fun, playful activity.

Bring a little flirtation back into your relationship by tacking it on to things you do already. Sure, it's sweet of you to bring him a cup of coffee in the morning. Make it a little salty by looking into his eyes, holding his gaze for a second and giving him a flirty smile as you hand it to him. Yes, she really does love an appreciative verbal thank you for doing the dishes. You'll stir more than her appreciation, however, if the thank you is delivered with a playful comment about how she looks almost as good doing them as she does doing you.

Good flirting is all about subtlety. If you come on too strong or you're trying too hard, it usually backfires and leaves your partner feeling turned off rather than turned on. You want sexy, not sleazy. Think more George Clooney, less drunk guy coming on to you at a party.

Regularly flirting with your partner will make them feel sexy and desirable. It will make you both more playful, and it'll maintain that twinkle in your relationship's eye. That's worth a bit of your time every day, isn't it?

TIME to PLAY

Five Minutes or Less

Mmm . . . Thinking of You

You're already texting, emailing and twittering all day, so take a minute to send your partner a sexy, flirty message. Utter a sexy "Mmm . . ." before a quick "thinking of you" voicemail, or add a few suggestive question marks to the note on the fridge telling her you plan on bringing home something "extra special" for dessert tonight. Send him a text in the middle of the day that says "Just had a sexy image pop into my head that I'd like to share with you later."

Feeling the Connection

When you're out with a group of people, run your hand down his arm or discreetly scratch her back as if to say "Hey baby, I'm so aware of you, even amongst all these people." When you're out together at a party, flash a wink across the room. When you're watching TV together, look over at her, make eye contact and give her a knowing smile.

You're Smokin', Baby

Any comments about how smokin', gorgeous, etc. your partner is are always welcome.

Imagine if you saw her across the room in a bar or at a party. What would strike you about her appearance? Tell her. *But she knows I think she's sexy,* you say with a shrug. She wants to hear it anyway. Telling her she's sexy and beautiful will feed the sexy and beautiful part of her, make her want to act on it and get you laid more regularly.

DM her on Twitter and describe what you find sexy about her in 140 characters. Get into the habit of sending her a daily email compliment. Was it how soft her lips were when she kissed you goodbye this morning? Did you love how her legs looked in that dress she wore? Be detailed. Telling her she looks nice is, well, nice. Be more specific: "You look great in green, hon, it really shows off your gorgeous eyes."

He loves sexy compliments too. If you don't believe me, watch his chest swell ever so slightly when you're out together and you lean over to whisper in his ear that he looks really hot tonight. Watch his eyes light up when he walks downstairs freshly showered and dressed and you eyeball him up and down, give him a sly smile and tell him you wish you didn't have to go to work because he looks *guuuhhhð*.

One Hour or Less
And You Are . . . ?
Meet at a bar after work and pretend you've never met. Use different names and let him try to pick you up. Or vice versa.

The Silent Treatment
Make a rule when you're out together socially one night that you can't speak to one another for an hour. The only way you can communicate is through body language. See where the conversation goes.

Contact Sport
During your next dinner conversation, add a physical gesture to everything you say to your sweetheart, no matter how mundane. Touch her cheek when you ask about her day. Brush your hand along his forearm as you tell him that you have a busy week ahead of you and will probably have to stay late at work several evenings.

All Night
Word Play
Play a game while you're out. Every time one of you gets up to go to the bathroom or get a drink, you have to whisper one sexy thing into the other person's ear before you go. Example: "Imagine my hot breath on your neck." Make it clear up front that you don't have to actually act on the suggestion. This is about awakening your sexual selves, opening up to each other and stirring desire.

Send Electronic Sparks
Start a flirtatious email or text conversation in the morning. Start with something like "Hey gorgeous, if I met you at a dinner party for the first time, what would you say to me if I said hello?" "I'd ask you if you always had such sexy dimples." Keep it going back and forth for as long as you can throughout the day.

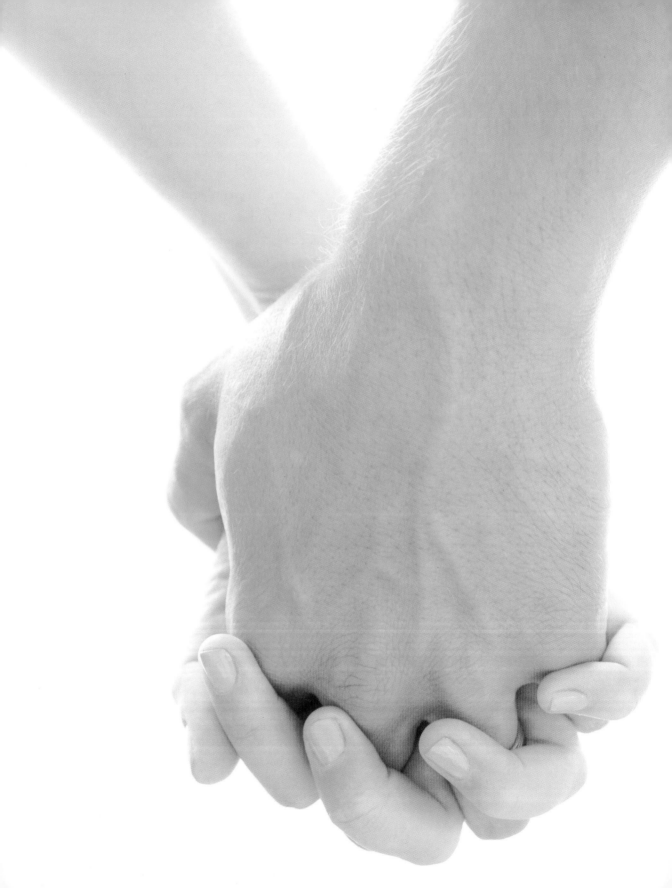

Chapter Three
DATE

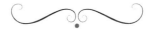

I'd like to reintroduce another favourite from the glory days of your courtship—the date. If you guys don't date anymore, you need to start. Dating is crucial if you want to keep the spark in your relationship, especially if you have kids. It's far too easy to settle into a relationship and get caught up in your daily routine. Your days are hectic and sometimes getting through them is all you can manage, but don't forget to schedule special time for just the two of you. If you don't plan any focused one-on-one time together, your relationship will suffer. It's as simple as that. Dates force you to stop and take notice of one another. They remind you of why you're together and what you love about being in one another's company. Best of all, dates are fun! Do you remember what it's like to have fun together?

If a night of fun together isn't enough motivation to get out for a special night, make a date, literally. Sit down with your smartphones, compare iCals and figure out a night that works for both of you. Then book it! Make a point of scheduling at least one full date night a month. I can hear you now: *Scheduling a date night isn't very romantic.* Let's examine that objection, shall we? In the early days of your relationship, I'm sure you didn't just coincidentally show up at the same restaurant or movie together. You planned it ahead of time, which gave you time to look forward to it. You probably spent some mental energy imagining how the night would go, put some thought into what you would wear, maybe got your nails done or put on a clean shirt. Scheduling a date isn't unromantic, it's exciting. Think of it as something to look forward to and you'll be more motivated to do it. Play the night in your head, think about what you're going to wear, plan something special for the evening—all the things that build anticipation, the fuel needed to keep desire alive.

Just because you've hooked each other permanently now, don't deny yourselves this pleasure. And as a permanent couple, you have an added advantage. When you were single and dating you had to play the odds by getting to know some stranger you might or might not like. The two of you presumably like each other, so you don't have to worry that your date's going to turn out to be a creep.

Dating gives you one-on-one time with your partner. Don't waste it talking about the kids or whether you have the money to fix the doohickey on the whichamabob. If you haven't had any face time with each other in a while, this could be a tempting opportunity to dump all the unspoken crap that's been building up between you. Not the time. On dates, keep the mood positive and leave the criticisms at home. Use dates as an opportunity to stimulate each other's minds. Remember, you're both adults with your own opinions, observations and stories to tell.

Think of dates as opportunities to remind your partner why they chose to be with you over everyone else in the world. Yes, think about that for a moment: Your partner picked *you* over everyone else in the world. Surely they deserve a bit of your undivided attention once in a while to assure them they made the right choice?

A date doesn't have to be an elaborate, expensive all-night affair. When you don't have the time for a formal date, you can turn everyday activities into mini-dates by doing something as simple as dressing up for dinner. Instead of turning on the TV after dinner, go for a walk so you can just talk and enjoy each other's company. The important thing is to make time together, be it five minutes or five hours.

TIME to PLAY

Five Minutes or Less

Don't Sweat It

Silently watching a movie together after the kids have gone to bed doesn't exactly qualify as an official date. Then again, if that's already on the schedule for the evening, at least make it date-like by sitting snuggled together on the couch with a nice glass of wine and some fancy snacks. Lose the PJs or sweats and put on something a little more seductive. Yes, I know now that you're comfy in the relationship you should be able to relax at home in your flannel PJs and sweats, but when you have so little time to be intimate, why not take advantage of moments like these and at least make the pajamas silk or satin? Fellas, if you've never worn a pair of men's silk pajama bottoms, don't knock it until you've tried it. Silk pajamas make you feel sexier the second you put them on. Ask her for a pair for your next birthday.

Dress for Dinner

Brilliantly portrayed on the TV series *Mad Men*, in the 1960s, men and women "dressed" for after-work cocktails and dinner, and kids were seen and not heard. I'm not suggesting we bring back the sexism and repression of the era, but there is something to be said for designating some adult time so the two of you can reconnect at the end of the day. I also love the idea of dressing for dinner. Do your hair and makeup and put on a sexy dress and heels for dinner at home tonight. Underwear optional.

Pizza by Candlelight

If you don't have time to cook, order pizza or microwave a couple of frozen dinners, but serve the meal by candlelight on your best dishes with a nice bottle of wine . . . on a blanket on your living room floor.

One Hour or Less

Date in a Jar

Much like a "Job Jar" (except a lot more fun) is a "Date Jar." In fact, make "Create a Date Jar" your first date idea. Sit down for an hour together and come up with simple things you could do together without planning ahead, like "Go for a walk after dinner," "Look through photos from when we first started dating," or "Take turns reading a book out loud to each other." Write all your ideas on slips of paper and stuff them in a jar. Any time you have a spare hour, instead of turning on the computer or the TV, shove your hand into the Date Jar and do whatever it tells you.

Conversation Starter

In the early days of your romance, you talked into the wee hours. It seemed there was no end to the things you had to talk about—the meaning of life, love, your pasts, your future together, and whether Paris Hilton was the first sign of the decline of Western civilization or a subversive feminist icon. Now you find yourselves having the same conversations every night over dinner: How was your day? What time do the kids have to be picked up from soccer tomorrow? Is it time to flip the mattress again? There is certainly comfort in the familiar, and sharing the mundane details of your day-to-day life can be reassuring, even sweet. But come on, you need to bring some fresh material to the table once in a while. If you've both got nothing, get creative. Pretend you're Angelina Jolie and Brad Pitt and have the conversation you imagine they'd have over dinner in the adult wing of their mansion.

Replay Date

Reenact your first date. If you can't physically do this, recount it to one another in as much detail as you can remember. Where did you go? What did you wear? What were your first impressions (stick to the positive or funny stuff)? What were you thinking at the time but didn't share that your sweetie would love to hear now?

All Night

Adventure Seekers

Studies have shown that dates involving highly adventurous, even daring activities fire up feel-good chemicals in your brain like dopamine, making you feel more attracted to one another. So plan a date that will get your dopamine pumping. Ever been bungee jumping together? White-water rafting? Go-karting? Dumpster diving? Use your imagination.

Something on Your Mind?

Go to an art gallery or a museum together. Start your own two-person book club where you read the same book and talk about it. Individually come up with a topic or place you want to learn more about. Research each other's choices and plan a dinner date to discuss your findings.

Retro Romance

Schedule a romantic night at a drive-in. Go for sodas afterward (okay, I don't actually know what "sodas" are, but find a burger joint to share a burger and fries—make sure you get two straws for your milkshake). Complete the night with a long, hot goodnight kiss on the front doorstep.

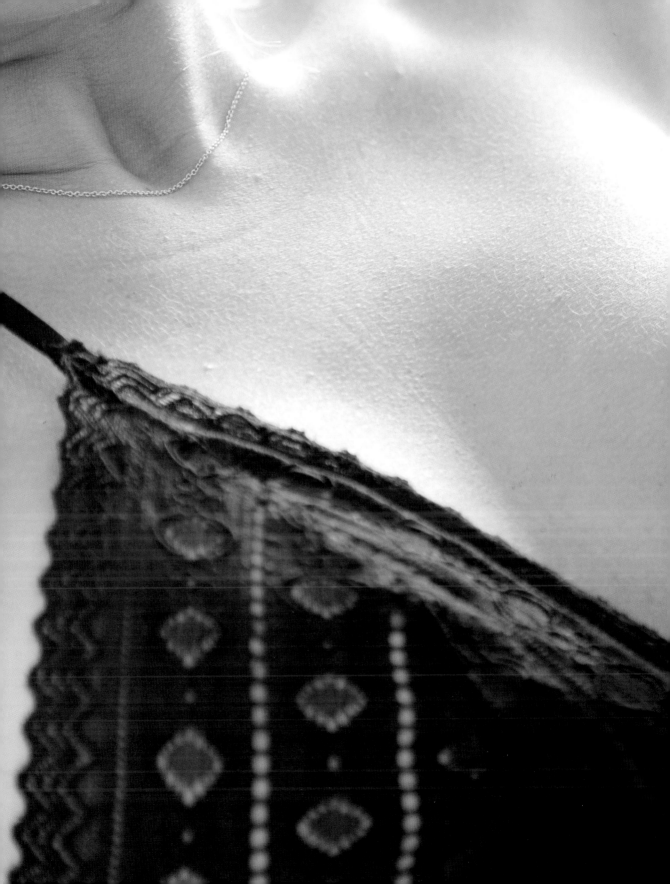

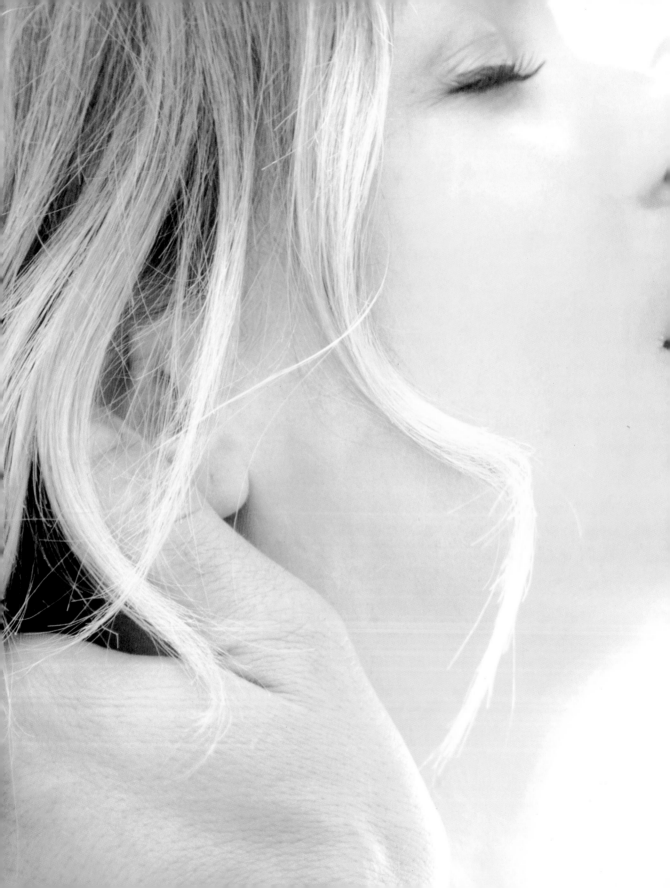

Chapter Four
KISS

I'm sure you remember vividly the first time the two of you kissed—that electric moment when your lips met, sealing an intimacy between you. Unfortunately, kissing often becomes automatic after you've been together for a while, be it a perfunctory kiss hello or goodbye or an obligatory step on the way to sex. What a shame to deprive yourselves of such a delicious activity, especially when you consider that your partner is the only person you get to kiss really deeply. Why would you not take advantage of this wonderful privilege every single day? It's time to rediscover the joys of smooching, to relish the feeling of pressing your mouths together to enjoy the warmth and softness of each other's lips. To imagine every kiss is your first.

Kissing also keeps you connected and intimate when there isn't time for sex. Think back to that great feeling when you were a teenager and sex wasn't an option yet. You necked until your lips were raw and you were in a fevered state. When you don't have time for sex, a great make-out session can keep you feeling hot for each other without having to get naked. In fact, when you consciously remove sex as an option (it's not like that possibility won't be around later if you're both interested), it forces you to get back to enjoying the intimate, sexy sensation of making out like a couple of teenagers (but with a lot more experience!). It may feel awkward at first, but keep at it and you'll awaken senses you forgot you had—senses you must nurture and tend if you want to keep desire on the front burner in your relationship.

TIME to PLAY

Five Minutes or Less

The Ten-Second Kiss

Kiss each other deeply at least once every day: before you leave in the morning, when you get home, while you're making dinner together or before you go to sleep (whether sex will follow or not). Make it last for at least ten seconds. Count it in your head. This may not feel very romantic, but counting will force you to stay with it because if

you're not used to doing this, ten seconds will feel like a long time at first. To do this at least once a day (though there's no rule you can't do it more frequently) requires less time than you spend brushing your teeth. Yet ten seconds of deep kissing daily will do a heck of a lot more to keep your relationship sexually charged and intimate than brushing your teeth. Keep things unpredictable by surprising one another with your kisses. When she's standing talking on the phone in her bathrobe, drop to your knees and plant kisses up and down her legs. If you're having a drink together, suck an ice cube into your mouth, then lean over and kiss him while passing the cold, wet ice between your mouths.

- - - - - - - - - - - - - - - - - -

Quick Tip:
Handy Trick

Practise kissing on your hand (c'mon, I bet you did it as a kid). Hold your hand palm down in front of you and kiss the back of it right behind the knuckle of your index finger.

- - - - - - - - - - - - - - - - - -

Plant a Hollywood Kiss

You've seen her melt as she watches her favourite leading man lean in to kiss his leading lady for the first time. Make her swoon with your most romantic silver-screen-worthy kiss. Ham it up for full effect. Gingerly brush her hair back off her face, look deeply into her eyes and smile. Brush your lips lightly across her eyebrow. Plant a few light kisses across her forehead. As you lean in to kiss her mouth, pause before your lips meet to build the anticipation. When she moves in to meet your kiss, pull back. Make her wait for it. Cup your hand behind her head to give the impending kiss a sense of dramatic urgency and, when the moment is right, lean in, close your eyes and press your relaxed, slightly parted lips against hers to kiss her fully for several seconds. Feel the connection between you. Open your eyes and look deeply into hers as you kiss. It may feel a little cheesy romantic-comedy at first, but it will intensify your connection with practice. When you finally pull away, look deep into her eyes again, caress her cheek and say, "Here's looking at you, kid." Or not, unless you're actually Humphrey Bogart. Stick to what feels most natural to you. End your kiss with a warm smile and a simple "I love you so much, baby."

A Little Bit of Heaven

Revisit that teen favourite Seven Minutes in Heaven but change it to Two Minutes in Heaven (c'mon, when you were young, you probably spent the first five minutes in awkward silence before anyone made a move anyway, right?) with the two of you the only players. Whenever one of you gets the urge (or every time the cat coughs up a hairball, if you need an outside trigger), yell, "Two Minutes in Heaven!" Then the two of you have to get into the closet together (pick one that's not full of, say, stinky gym equipment) and make out for a full two minutes, above the belt.

Quick Tip:
Whisper Naughty Somethings

While you're making out, brush your lips across his ear and, in your sexiest raspy voice, tell him how hot his kisses are making you.

One Hour or Less

French Connection

Your first kiss "with tongue" was serious business. It was like the gateway drug to sex. As an adult, adding tongue to your kisses can also be sexy if done with caution. Too much tongue before she's ready for it can be off-putting. Get her warmed up first with plenty of regular kissing. Introduce your tongue to other areas before introducing it to her mouth. Run a light tongue along her neck or in behind her earlobe. Take her finger in your mouth and let her watch you swirl your wet, soft tongue all around it. Slide your tongue across her bottom lip. Gauge her reaction. If she tenses up, it might be too soon for tongue. If she enjoys it, gently slide the tip of your tongue between her slightly parted lips. Go back to regular kissing for a moment. When it feels right, slip your tongue into her mouth. Think less darting snake or slobbery cow, more sexily licking your fingers after eating a messy rack of BBQ ribs. If she's responsive and meets your tongue with her own, swirl the firm tip of your tongue around hers. Quickly suck her tongue into your mouth once or twice to turn up the heat. Then go back to kissing. Once you get your tongue involved it doesn't have to remain on the scene. Less is more. Use it to create more intensity, then pull back and return to kissing with your mouth. Keep her hungry for you.

Sink Your Teeth into It

If you ever had a hickey when you were a teenager, you know the excitement of surrendering yourself to that wonderful shivery feeling of someone sucking passionately on your neck to the point of causing internal bleeding. No adult wants to spend the next week in turtlenecks or telling lies involving curling irons, but you can still use your teeth to tap into that wonderful threshold between pain and pleasure—without the internal bleeding. Use your teeth to convey urgency, like you want to eat him up. As with your tongue, use your teeth sparingly and strategically to introduce a bit of naughtiness to your kisses. An unexpected nibble between kisses introduces an edgy sense of danger that's exhilarating and arousing. When he's pulling away from a kiss, grab hold of his bottom lip between your teeth and gently bite down before you let him go. If his tongue is in your mouth, hold it gingerly between your teeth and let them scrape lightly along the sides of his tongue as he pulls it out of your mouth. Plant a series of gentle nibbles along his neck. Take his earlobe into your mouth, lightly bite down and graze your teeth along it as you pull your mouth away.

Simon Says . . . Kiss Me

Obviously, kissing is subjective and, while there are general guidelines you can follow, the best way to know how your partner

---

Quick Tip: Feel the Pull

If she pulls away or seems uncomfortable at any time, sloooow down. Sighs and moans are usually a sign you're doing something right. Pull back and let her lead once in a while so she gets a chance to control the action. Occasionally pull back or lighten up your kisses to leave her wanting more.

---

likes to be kissed is to have them tell you. Or, even better, demonstrate. This can be both instructional and hot. Take turns describing in detail one type of kiss you would enjoy. Back up your instruction with a little demo, kissing your partner the way you've just described. Have them show you what they learned. Now switch.

All Night

Make It a Date

If you can't find time for regular make-out sessions in your routine, schedule a kissing date—no sex allowed. Get together somewhere where sex isn't an option so you have to keep things above the belt, like a park bench (pretend you're in Paris).

Park It

I grew up in the country, where "parking" was a great teenage pastime. When you were a teenager, finding a time and place to make out without getting caught was a challenge. The sneaky nature of the act made the whole thing so steamy. Inject some of this thrill into your relationship. On your way home from dinner, make a detour onto a dead-end street and "park," keeping the action neck-up only.

Keep Your Mouth Shut

Email your sweetie an invite to a "no-kissing-on-the-lips" date in your bedroom that night. Two rules: No kissing on the lips and no sex. Kiss each other anywhere but on the lips . . . earlobe, neck, shoulder, inside the elbow, along the calf.

Quick Tip:
Room for Improvement

If you don't like the way your partner kisses, stopping him in the middle and telling him he's a lousy kisser will not likely improve the situation. Instead, try this:

- If his kisses are too hard, for example, simply stop him, hold his face and gently, using your most seductive voice, ask him to kiss you as lightly and slowly as he can.

- If you're watching a romantic movie together and like a particular screen kiss, tell him you find it extremely hot and would love the two of you to try kissing like that.

- Suggest trying different types of kisses—soft, hard, with tongue, etc.—and gently comment on what you like and don't like about each other's technique.

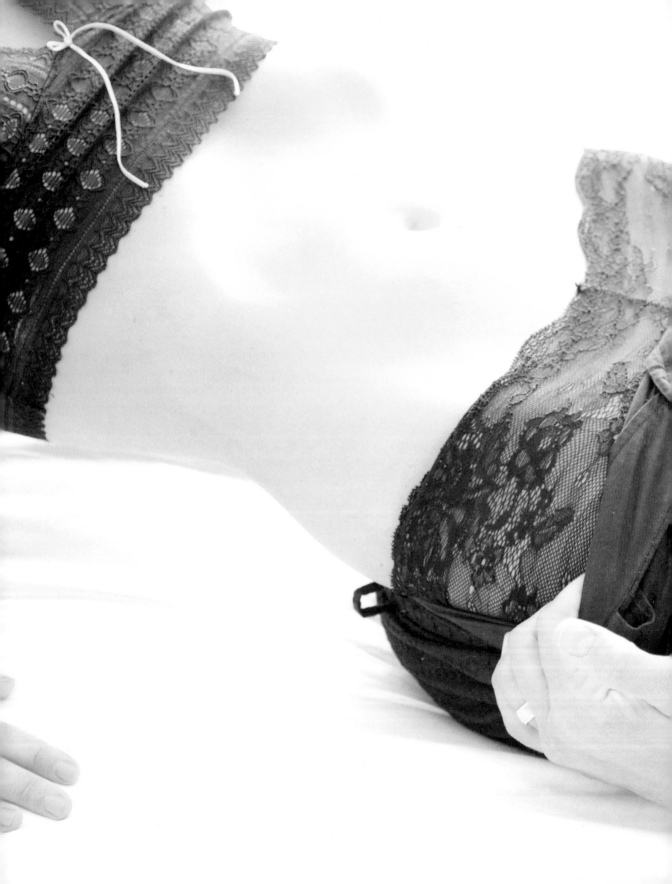

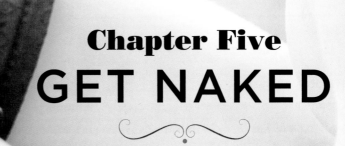

Chapter Five
GET NAKED

The first time you saw each other naked, you couldn't believe your good fortune. What a privilege and an honour it was that your partner was literally and figuratively exposing themselves to you. By now you've seen each other naked so many times, you barely think about it. With familiarity, the intimacy of seeing each other naked loses its sexual charge. Which simply won't do if you're trying to keep desire alive and well. So let's put the fun and excitement back into getting naked and turn the every-day act of getting undressed back into an event that gets you noticing each other again. Build anticipation by putting plenty of tease into peeling each other's clothes off, keeping in mind that slow is good and slower is better. If you're shy about being in the buff, use it. Acting coy is the perfect tease that says "What, me? Naughty? Never. Okay, maybe just a little peek."

Taking your clothes off isn't open-heart surgery, so don't take it too seriously and keep things playful and flirty. I know we all have our body issues, but keep in mind that a less-than-perfect body carried with confidence is hotter than a flawless body carried self-consciously. If you believe in what you're selling, your partner will buy it. If you're still nervous, some red lighting (think scarves over the lamps or coloured light bulbs) or candlelight will definitely help with the presentation.

TIME to PLAY

Five Minutes or Less
Secret Exhibit
You don't need to put on an elaborate striptease to tap into your inner exhibitionist. Whisper in his ear over a dinner date that you're not wearing any underwear.

Bedtime Beefcake
When you're getting ready for bed, playfully show her some of your best cheesy Chippendale dancer moves as you change into your PJs.

Flash Pants
Invest in a pair of stockings and a garter belt. Wear them with high heels and let your skirt slide up so he gets a glimpse of the garter strap when you cross your legs in the taxi on the way to a party. Or wear some sexy underwear under your work clothes and flash him before you leave in the morning so that the image of you in your sexy undies stays with him all day.

One Hour or Less
Show Off
Tell him to go into your closet and pick out several outfits he finds sexy. Model each ensemble using your best fashion model strut. Then un-model each outfit for him.

Just Because You're Naked Doesn't Mean You Have to Have Sex
Get naked and enjoy each other's bodies without going all the way. Have a warm, sudsy, slippery bubble bath together. If you have the privacy, sunbathe in the nude together, letting the sun's rays pour down on your genitals and breasts. (Just don't stay out too long. You definitely do not want to burn your delicate bits.) Nude wrestling? Why not? Throw down a plastic sheet (use a shower curtain) and oil each other up to make it really interesting. Or if you've never eaten a sundae off your partner's tummy, what are you waiting for?

Not Baring It All
Sometimes leaving a little something to the imagination is just as much, or more, of a turn-on as being naked. Watching you

strut around in a pair of sexy undies and a lacy bra (granny pants and a stretched-out laundry-day bra might not have the best effect) leaves more to the imagination than seeing you naked. Wear a silky slip and slide yourself up and down his naked body. Have sex with your undies on and simply pulled to one side. Take your panties off but leave your skirt on and have sex with you on top. Wear a pair of high heels—and nothing else. It will make you feel sexy— taller, thinner and more confident.

Quick Tip:
Under Cover

If you're self-conscious about your breasts, wear a racy bra during sex. If you're self-conscious about your tummy, wear a sexy T-shirt and no bra. Not only does this help you stop worrying about what your body looks like, it also gives sex a fiery "we couldn't even wait to get our clothes off" urgency.

All Night

Tear Each Other's Clothes Off . . . Literally

Ripping each other's clothes off in the heat of passion certainly has its charm, though it could get expensive. If you're not keen to destroy your $500 Calvin Klein suit, hang on to some play clothes you don't care about so you can literally rip them off each other. Throw these on instead of some sweats when you get home from work as a non-verbal way of telling your partner to go for it.

Peel and Play

Take as long as you possibly can to undress her. In fact, take what you think is slow and multiply it by ten. The longer you take to peel each item of clothing from her, the more sexually worked up she'll get. It's all about the tease, baby. Take your sweet time with snaps and zippers. If she's wearing a shirt, undo it one agonizingly slow button at a time. Every time you expose some skin, spend time kissing it before moving on. As you undress her, tell her what you love about her body and compliment her on her best assets.

Now remove her shirt but leave her bra as you work your way down. If she's wearing a belt, unbuckle it slooowly. When it's unbuckled, grab both ends in one hand and use it to pull her toward you and give her a deep, long kiss. Slip your finger inside the waist of her pants or skirt and slide it back and forth a few times. Go back to kissing some exposed skin. Undo the button of her pants or skirt but leave the zipper done up. Briefly press your hand against her covered groin. Unzip her bit by bit. Slip your hand down the front of her pants or skirt and caress her through her underwear, just for a second or two. Drag your fingertips along the inside edge of her bra, letting your fingernails gently scratch the soft flesh of her breasts. Use your mouth to kiss each bra strap off her shoulders and take your time undoing the clasp at the back. If you can't get her damn bra unhooked, who cares? Ask her to unhook it for you and then slowly lower each shoulder strap. As you slide them down her arms, caress the sides of her breasts. Run your tongue across each nipple. Trust me, she'll quickly forget any fumbling.

Pull off her bottoms inch by inch. Leave her underwear on and press your open mouth against it so she can feel your warm breath through the fabric. Take your time with her panties, kissing her thighs and calves as you shimmy them down her legs. Now take a moment to let her know how much you enjoy the view before you eat her up . . . or whatever it is you choose to do next. Nice work, tiger!

Show Time

Most women have fantasized about stripping for their partner. And most men have fantasized about having their partner strip for them. Which works out rather nicely. A striptease can happen spontaneously, if the mood and the opportunity strike. But it can also be fun to put some extra effort into making it a special occasion. Send him an invite, whether by email, text or a heart-shaped note on his pillow, telling him that you'd like him to attend a special private show at a certain date and time.

> 66 Striptease is all about anticipation. Remove each article of clothing slowly, slowly, slowly. The longer you drag it out, the more it will drive him crazy. 99

Just before show time, get yourself in the mood. Have a bath while enjoying a glass of wine to ease any nerves (just don't get too relaxed, you don't want to fall off your stilettos). The traditional stockings, garter, sexy bra and underwear and high heels combo is always a sure winner, but a silky negligee, a slutty short skirt or a hot dress you know he loves will also do the trick. Whatever makes you feel sexy. The more layers, the longer the tease. That's not to say you should show up in a parka and seven sweaters, though that would have its own funny charm if you played it right. Think gloves that can be pulled off one delectable finger at a time or a shirt with lots of buttons or hooks.

Put on some music and pull up a comfy chair for your audience (one with arms is great because you can use it to perch a high heel on or to support your hands as you wiggle your bum in his face or his lap should you choose). Chill some champagne. Dim the lamps and light some candles. Slip on a robe (satin is sexier than terrycloth), pour yourself a glass of bubbly and wait for your audience. When he arrives, let him take in the ambience while you pour him his beverage of choice and guide him to his seat. Lean over him and look him in the eyes, give him a deep kiss, make a toast and start the show.

As you stand facing him, let your robe casually fall open so he gets a hint of what's underneath and pull it closed again. Turn away and slip your robe off one shoulder as you look back at him, then let it drop to the floor as you walk away. Turn around and strut toward him. Use the chair arms to support yourself as you make your breasts sway in front of his face. Bend over at the waist and, as you straighten up, slide both hands, fingers spread, up your calves and along your inner thighs. Continue to move your hands up your body, running a finger around each nipple through your top with a look on your face that says "Mmm, this feels good, I bet you wish you were my hands right now." Striptease is all about anticipation and, duh, the tease. Remove each article of clothing slowly, slowly, slowly. The longer you drag it out, the more it will drive him crazy.

Once you've stripped down to your garters/stockings and heels, walk toward him, turn around and bend over at the waist to grab your ankles and swing your bottom right in front of his eyes. If you're self-conscious about your rear view, sit down on his lap instead, lay your body back against his and shimmy it up and down. By now, he should pretty much be at your mercy. Feel free to tease him some more. Or grab him by the hand, lead him to the bed and have your way with him.

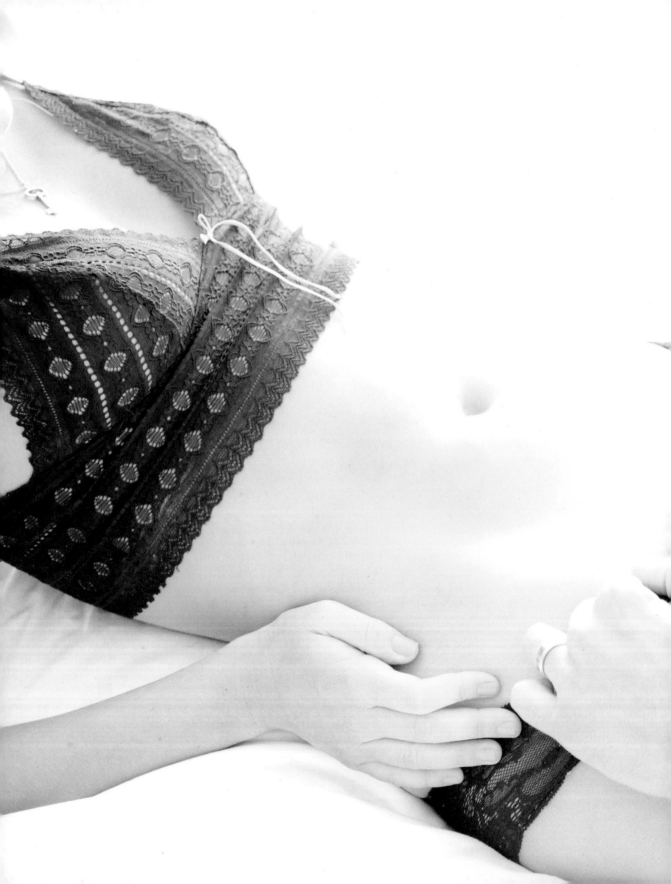

❧ Seduction Cheat Sheet ❧

☐ Send a text, email or voicemail message at least once a day that lets your partner know you're thinking of them.

☐ Add some spice to the occasional message to keep the spark alive.

☐ Compliment each other daily.

☐ Verbalize your appreciation for the things you both do for each other.

☐ Schedule at least one date night a month.

☐ Make time for adult conversation that doesn't include the house and kids.

☐ Kiss each other deeply for ten seconds at least once a day.

☐ Have regular no-sex make-out sessions.

☐ Make getting undressed an occasion.

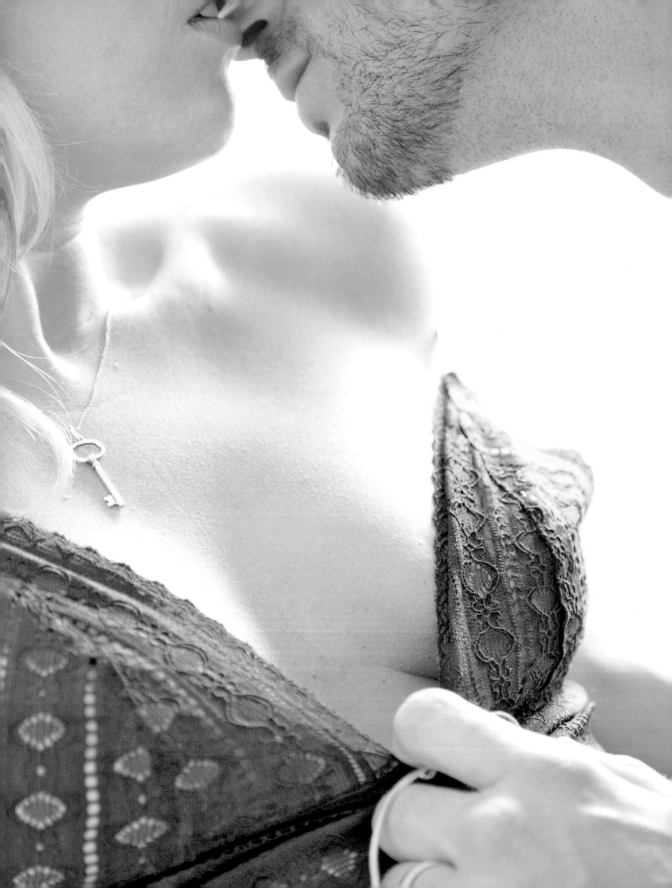

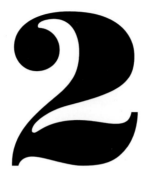

FOREPLAY

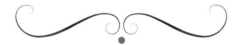

The word "foreplay" has always been a bit of an issue for me because it implies that any activity categorized within it is merely a pit stop be"fore" you get to the Main Event, that is, intercourse—the *real* sex. Frankly, I don't care if the stuff in this chapter happens 'fore, after or somewhere 'tween. I'd much prefer you focus on the latter part of the word—the "play" part. Because I think that sex—all aspects of it—should ultimately be fun. When something is fun, you look forward to it, and, that's right, you make time for it.

Also, whether foreplay is used as a warm-up for intercourse or is an event all on its own, you'll both look forward to it even more if you know what you're doing in this department. Because, let's be honest, if your guy gives lousy massage, you're hardly going to clear your calendar for it, are you? And if her blow jobs are a little, well, blah, you might not be so enthusiastic about rushing home for one, right? So let's solve two problems. Let's find time for more foreplay in your life and let's make your foreplay the best it can be!

Foreplay comes in many forms, so I cover a lot of ground. I start with the importance of non-sexual touch and how crucial it is for you to keep the connection between you alive by literally staying in touch with one another even, or especially, when you're not naked. Then there is the delicious form of touch that lies between the tender and the sexual: massage. I explain how to use massage to connect on a more sensual level and guide you step by step if you decide you'd like to give each other an extra-sensual massage, if you know what I mean. From there, we veer into the territory of self-pleasure for a minute because getting to know your own body through masturbation can help improve your sex life together, and also because incorporating masturbation itself into your lovemaking can be hot. Next stop, his and hers hand jobs, where you'll find lots of detailed instruction on how to handle one another in ways that will make you, well, unable to keep your hands off each other. I wrap up with some fine dining tips. The oral sex sections cover everything from improving your cunnilingus or fellatio technique to test-driving some new oral sex positions to answering the question I know has been burning in your brain: Do chin-strap dildos really work?

Time Challenge

If you have ten seconds . . .
Whisper one thing you'd like your partner to try next time they, um, handle you.

If you have thirty seconds . . .
Drop to your knees and give him ten slow licks while he's uncorking the wine for dinner.

If you have one minute . . .
Stop whatever you're doing and hug each other tightly for an entire minute.

If you have five minutes . . .
Set a timer and tell her to lie back and enjoy five solid minutes of non-reciprocal oral sex.

If you have ten minutes . . .
Ask him to let you watch him masturbate while you kiss and caress his body.

If you have fifteen minutes . . .
Give each other a foot massage.

If you have an hour . . .
Make a "no intercourse" rule and spend an hour pleasuring each other using hands only.

If you have all night . . .
Use scented candles, warm oil and soothing music and indulge her with a full-body massage complete with happy ending.

START WITH THE BASICS

Set the mood.

Light some candles, pour a glass of wine, lock the bedroom door.

Get comfy.

You'll enjoy whatever you're doing a whole lot more if you're both comfortable.

Practise good hygiene.

Make sure hands and nails are clean, and mouths and genitals are fresh.

Ease into it.

You'll get a better response from your partner if you warm them up.

Don't just touch, feel.

Touching is a monologue, feeling is a conversation. Every time you touch your partner, be conscious of the connection between you.

Tease.

Always leave your partner wanting more.

Be unpredictable without being too scattered.

Variety is welcome but not to the point of distraction.

Be enthusiastic.

Make your partner feel like there's nowhere else you'd rather be.

When in doubt, ask.

It'll save you driving around the block a few extra times.

Don't worry about the final destination.

Ironically, the more you pay attention to the route, rather than where you're going, the greater the chance you'll get there.

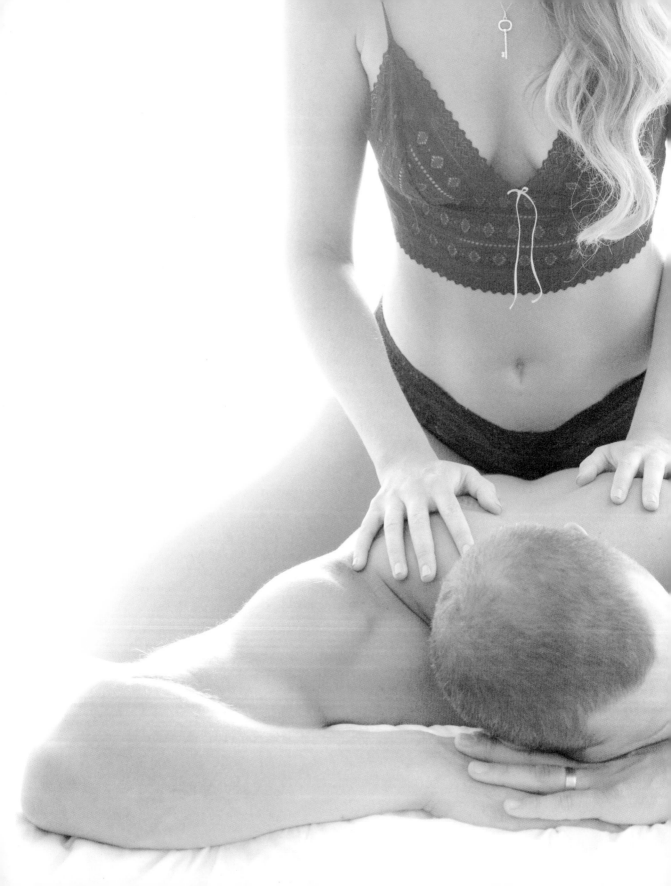

Chapter Six
TOUCH

The knowledge that your partner understands exactly how to touch you in all the right ways has benefits beyond the obvious pleasure in the moment. The mere thought of her touch can do wonders for getting you through a dull office meeting. And I'm not referring only to sexual touch. Knowing how to touch your partner in a non-sexual way is equally important. Women often complain to me that the only time their guy really touches them in a meaningful way is when he wants to have sex. Be sure to touch her in ways that aren't overtly sexual. When you're strapped for time and feeling disconnected, just the feel of your partner's hand in yours can keep you literally and emotionally connected. Whenever you're together, make a point of caressing her cheek, rubbing her temples or running your hand across her lower back.

Whether your touch is sexual or not, make sure there is meaning behind it. You want her to feel like touching her is all you want to do, that you can't help yourself. Rather than simply saying the words "I love you," take a moment to hold her hand between yours, look her in the eyes and say it. It only takes a second or two longer but adds extra meaning to your words by making her feel that you're truly present. Ironically, this non-sexual touch will ultimately make her more sexually open to you. Honest.

The deal runs both ways. He wants to feel your touch beyond the bedroom. Run your fingers through his hair while you're watching TV and tell him how much you love him. Rub your hands across his shoulders and down his upper arms after he's had a long day at work. Scratch his back. Give his butt a squeeze or slide your hand into his while you're out at a party together.

When you don't have time for more elaborate sexual play, daily touch is essential to sustain intimacy. It takes a second to put your arm around her while you're watching your kids' hockey game. When you're riding silently together in the car, brushing your hand along his thigh and giving it a squeeze while he's driving says "I may be lost in my own thoughts but you're never far from them." That said, it's also essential that you know how to

touch your partner in more sensual ways. Too often, when couples get sexual, they forget to keep touching and really feeling each other. Massage is an excellent way to practise touching your partner more sensually. When you massage your partner, you can pay closer attention to responses and use the opportunity to discover previously uncharted sensitive areas. The other great thing about massage is that it can be either PG or X-rated, making it an excellent broker between non-sexual and sexual touch. It can also take as little or as much time as you have, from a quick shoulder or foot rub to an evening of relaxing full-body massage complete with happy ending. And unless your partner has serious issues with feeling relaxed and pampered, they are not going to say no to a massage, no matter how little time they have.

Don't believe me? Try it. Ask her right now if she'd like you to rub her shoulders. See?

TIME to PLAY

Five Minutes or Less

Hand It Over

Whenever I see an elderly couple walking down the street holding hands, it makes my heart swell. *Now there's a couple that's still in love,* I think. I'm sure that, early in the relationship, you held hands all the time without even thinking about it. If you've stopped, reintroduce this simple and romantic gesture. Grab hold of your sweetie's hand and give it a squeeze while you're walking down the street together. Make it a regular habit and you too will end up being that old couple that everyone envies.

Hug It Out

Hugging is a powerful way to stay emotionally and physically connected through non-sexual touch. In fact, research shows that hugs release oxytocin, the bonding chemical. After you both get home from work and are in the midst of rushing around getting dinner ready and the kids organized, make a point of stopping and holding each other for an entire minute. Set the stove timer and stay with it for the entire minute, melding into each other and really feeling the connection. If a minute feels too long at first, start with a ten-second hug and work your way up, extending the hug for five seconds every day.

Mini Massage

Give her a one-minute neck massage while she's sitting at the kitchen table enjoying her morning coffee. Walk up behind her, pull her hair aside and lightly kiss her neck. Rub your hands together to warm them and wrap your flat hands loosely around her neck. Using some pressure (but not too much), slide your hands down either side of her neck and out to each shoulder. Repeat this move five times, imagining yourself pulling the tension from her neck right out through her shoulders.

> 66 Walk up behind her, pull her hair aside and lightly kiss her neck. 99

Take five minutes when he gets home from work and get him to lie on the bed while you sit on his bum with your knees resting on either side of his body. Blow on your hands to warm them. Place your thumbs on either side of his spine and firmly run them down the entire length of his back. Lay a flat hand on either side of his spine, thumbs pointed toward it. Applying pressure with your fingertips, your thumbs and the heels of your hands (the firm part of your palm where your hand meets your wrist), move your hands out from the centre of his back. Repeat this stroke as you move down the entire length of his back.

One Hour or Less

The Multi-task Massage

Giving your partner a foot or head massage while you're lying on the couch watching TV makes wasting time together so much more enjoyable. Get him to lay his head in your lap and rub circles around his temples using your middle and index fingers, gently applying a bit of pressure as you rub. Use the fingertips of both hands to massage his scalp, repeatedly moving from the front of his head to the back. Take her socks off and lay her feet in your lap. Place your thumb on the top of her foot and your forefinger on the bottom and, squeezing gently, wiggle your way to the end of her big toe. Repeat this with each toe of each foot.

Couple Massage

Getting a massage from your partner is an intimate and welcome treat. However, when you're both stressed and tight for time, the job may be best left to the professionals. Plenty of spas offer couple massages so you can both go and get a massage at the same time in the same room. It can not end the way a full-body massage can end at home, but you do get to lie there and listen to each other ooh and aah without having to lift a finger.

Below the Belt

Get the blood flowing throughout her genital region by massaging her thighs, hips and bum. Have her lie on the bed on her back wearing her underwear or a pair of loose pajama pants. Wrap both hands around the upper thigh of one leg and slide them down the length of her thigh, squeezing your hands together and pressing your thumbs into her thigh as you do. Slide like this several times down one thigh, then switch legs and repeat. Wrap your hands around her hips, fingers splayed and thumbs pointed inward and lying flat on each hip. Press your thumbs gently into each hip and move them in circles around the entire hip area. Have her roll over and use the same technique on her buttocks, hands flat, fingers spread, thumbs making circles as you move around each cheek. Avoid any direct genital contact unless she encourages it. The main idea here is to get the blood flowing and awaken her sexual energy. She gets to decide if she wants to do anything about it. No pressure. I mean it.

All Night

Sexy Spa Date

It can be challenging to find time for a full-body massage. So make time. Tell her you want to schedule a "spa" appointment, just as she would book a hair appointment or a pedicure. Plan for at least a couple of hours when you can be alone, undisturbed. Arrange child care if necessary. If you like, give her a hint of what's to come, so to speak, by telling her you'd like to book a "sexy spa" appointment or a "spa with benefits." That way, she can put herself in a more sensual frame of mind for it. Just don't assume that her accepting your invite gives you the green light to go all the way. But let's not get ahead of ourselves.

Start the evening by having her relax in the tub with a glass of wine while you get set up. Create a relaxing, soothing and romantic atmosphere in the room: Unplug the phone, turn off all mobile devices, light some candles, put on some relaxing music and make sure the room is nice and warm so you'll both be comfy. Wear a bathrobe or some loose cotton pants and a T-shirt and, if you're using massage oil, throw some old towels or an old bedspread on the bed to protect your linens. Once you're ready, tell her to towel off, slip on a robe and join you. Then remove her robe and ask her to lie down on her stomach. If she prefers to keep her underwear on, that's fine—the less self-conscious she is, the more relaxed she'll be. Place a large, fluffy towel over her and uncover just the parts you are massaging, at least until you're both warmed up. How naked you both end up will depend on how things go.

If you're giving her a massage on the bed, you'll find it easiest to start by kneeling and straddling her back. Rub your hands together vigorously to warm and energize them. It may be funny to plop your ice-cold feet on your partner in bed in the middle of winter to make her jump out of her socks, but that's not the effect you're going for

here. Pour some oil into your hands and rub them together to warm it before applying to her body. If you want to drip oil directly onto her skin, warm it up (just make sure it's not too hot!) by putting the container in a bowl of hot water before you start.

You may feel like you're not very good at giving a massage, but don't worry too much about getting it right, especially at first. As with any kind of intimate touch, it takes time to figure out what works for your partner. Do keep in mind that the difference between a sensual massage and a regular "please pummel that pinched nerve out of its misery now" one is that sensual massage is more about pleasure than pain. Be firm, but not too firm. No pummelling . . . or pinching or pounding. Beyond that basic rule, here are a few specific things you can try:

• Use upward strokes with flat hands, palms down. Use the heels of your hands and/or your thumbs to add pressure as you stroke.

• Squeeze your partner's flesh between thumb and fingertips, release and repeat, as if kneading dough, being very careful not to press too hard. Think kneading, not pinching.

• Drag your fingertips lightly across her skin, letting them dance across the surface.

• Press just your fingertips, either together or slightly spread, into her flesh, sliding as you press. Do the same thing using circular motions.

• Make a fist and slide it along as you wiggle the knuckles back and forth into her flesh.

AT YOUR FINGERTIPS

Large, fluffy towel

Scented massage oil

Candles

Relaxing music

Old sheet or towels

Finally, don't rush through it. Spend several minutes working an area—repeating strokes, trying different ones—before moving on. Add more oil as needed. Be conscious of the energy flowing from your hands and fingertips into her skin and throughout her body as you massage her. Imagine an electric current vibrating between your skin and hers as you slide both hands up her back or press your fingertips into her shoulders.

If you've ever gone for a professional massage, you'll notice they work your body quite systematically, usually starting with the back and shoulders and moving on to your arms and legs. Then you roll over and they massage the front of your legs and arms and end with the neck, temples and head. You don't have to follow the same order, but some sort of routine is more relaxing than having your body parts massaged randomly. Here is a basic routine to get you started:

Begin with her neck and shoulders. Place your hands flat on either side of her neck, fingers spread, thumbs resting on the back of her neck. Slide your hands down, across the tops of her shoulders and down her upper arms, squeezing gently with your fingers and thumbs as you do (check in with her on occasion to gauge if

---

Quick Tip: Like This?

Pay attention to your partner's body language. If she tenses up, she's telling you she's not a fan of what you're doing. It may be that you're using too much pressure or you're touching an area she's particularly sensitive about. Ease up or back off and move your hands somewhere else. If she relaxes again, you've understood. If her body jerks or flinches, it may be that your touch is too light and ticklish. If you're not sure, ask for feedback. Don't disturb the peace with a lot of distracting chatter. Simple yes-or-no questions like "Harder?" or "Softer?" or "Do you not like that part of your body touched?" should be enough to help you out.

the pressure is too hard or too soft). Grasp her shoulders and press your thumbs into her shoulder blades, sliding your thumbs in a circular motion. Make fists and wiggle your knuckles back and forth across her shoulder blades and down her upper back. Place the heels of your hands against her shoulder blades, pushing down as you slide outward or in circles across her back and shoulders.

> 66Imagine an electric current vibrating between your skin and hers as you slide both hands up her back or press your fingertips into her shoulders.99

Next, spread your fingers and run them firmly down the length of each of her arms. Imagine pulling her stress and tension down her arms and out her fingertips. Cup one of her hands, palm facing up, in both of yours and press your thumbs into her palm. Slide your thumb from her palm up along her fingers, squeezing and wiggling each one between your thumb and forefinger as you imagine pulling the tension out through her fingertips.

Make a loose fist with each hand. Position your fists knuckles down and use me-dium pressure to wiggle them along either side of her spine from the nape of her neck right down to the top of her butt. Slide back up by pressing the flat tips of your thumbs on either side of her spine. Move up and down her spine like this several times as you imagine the energy flowing up and down her body.

Quick Tip:
Positive Reinforcement
If you know your partner is self-conscious about certain body parts, spend extra time massaging these areas while telling her how much you love them and how beautiful they are. This will create a more positive body/mind association and help overcome any anxiety about being naked.

Now, stand or kneel beside her, place both hands on the back of one leg and knead your way down the back of her thigh and all the way down her calf. Repeat with the other leg. Stand at the end of the bed and cradle one shin in your hands while kneading her calf with your thumbs all the way down to her ankles. Continue along her foot, wiggling your fingers and thumbs along the length of her foot (if her feet are ticklish, press your thumbs harder into the bottoms of them as you wiggle along). When you get to her toes, grasp each one between your thumb and forefinger and imagine drawing the tension out as you slide from the base to the tip of each little piggie.

> 66If you have all night, why not use it to turn up the heat on your massage?99

Once you've spent as much time as you like on her backside, quietly ask her to turn over, and focus on the front of her body. Place a towel or blanket across her pelvic area to keep her warm and to send the message that you intend to keep things clean for now. This will help her relax if she doesn't want to go there and build anticipation if she does. She may want a towel over her breasts as well. Check with her to see what she prefers.

Start with her lower body. Standing or kneeling beside her, place both hands on one thigh and knead your way down the length of her leg several times. Repeat with the other leg. Kneel or stand at the foot of the bed, lean forward and wrap both hands around the top of one leg. Twist your hands back and forth down the entire length of her leg, pressing your thumbs into her flesh as you work your way all the way down to her feet and toes. Squeeze each toe between your finger and thumb and wiggle your way to the tip as you imagine pulling the tension out of her entire body through her toes.

> 66Imagine pulling the tension out of her entire body.99

Finish with her neck and head. Position yourself so that you're sitting or standing facing the top of her head and cradle it in one hand. Slide the other hand, fingers spread, up and down the back of her neck, pausing at the base to knead it with your fingertips. Switch hands and repeat, and then gently return her head to the bed. Position your fingertips above her eyebrows and drag them back along her forehead and

Quick Tip: Good Timing

Have a clock or timer in the room and tell her beforehand the duration of the massage (fifteen to sixty minutes, depending on your stamina). Knowing you're committed to a set amount of time will help her to relax and not worry that you might be tired or that the massage has gone on too long.

down through her hair to draw the tension out through the top of her head. Repeat several times. Finish with a gentle kiss on her forehead.

Those are some ideas for a basic PG massage. That might be all she wants tonight. Of course, if you have all night, why not use it to turn up the heat on your massage? Just as an option. As I mentioned earlier, even if you framed this evening as a sexy spa night, it's important that you still give her the choice if, in the end, she wants to keep things PG. You'll undo the good you've done if you push things too quickly without testing the waters first. How do you do this? When things get heated up to the point where you think you'd like to try and turn your sensual massage into a sexual massage, you could simply ask her if she wants you to go further. If she nods or groans, then yes, by all means. If you don't want to interrupt the flow with verbal communication, try this:

Once you've given her the full-body treatment and she's still lying on her back, start massaging her thighs. After a few minutes, slide the back of your hand all the way up the inside of her thigh, barely brushing the space between her legs before sliding the back of your hand down the inside of her other thigh. If she tenses up or closes her thighs, she's telling you she doesn't want you to go there. Go back to massag-

ing her legs, back and shoulders to let her know you get the message. If, however, she relaxes further (perhaps even spreading her thighs to give you better access) and lets out a "yes, that feels amazing" moan, she's telling you she's open to sexual touch. Continue this stroke, sliding the back of your hand up the inside of one thigh, across her sweet spot and back down the inside of her other thigh, pressing the back of your hand more firmly with each subsequent stroke. Trail your fingertips through her pubic hair (or the area where pubic hair once lived if she's clean-shaven), over her tummy and across each breast, grazing her nipples along the way.

Quick Tip:
I Surrender

As the massage recipient, surrender to his touch and use the opportunity to relax and bask in the sensations your body is feeling.

Now that she is nicely turned on, kneel, straddling her thighs. Oil up your hands and place each one flat on the top of each of her thighs, fingers spread, thumbs pointing toward the Promised Land. Press your thumbs into the crevice where her inner thigh meets her outer labia and slide them all the way down the crease and back up again. Repeat this stroke several times. As her arousal builds, inch your thumbs closer together with each upward stroke. Every few strokes, allow the flat of each thumb to slide across her clitoris one after the other. If she's moaning her appreciation, feel free to make some noise of your own. Deep breaths with each stroke will communicate your rising excitement. Let out a soft, meaningful, breathy "Mmm" to let her know how good this feels (and looks) to you.

> **"If she's moaning her appreciation, feel free to make some noise of your own."**

Once you've established deep relaxation along with heightened sexual arousal, you can decide where and how far to take it. You may both decide you want to take this sexual energy into intercourse. Or you could "massage" her to orgasm. For help with this, see "Hand Job for Her" on page 74. If you feel her getting frustrated or distracted, she probably isn't going to get there, but don't sweat it. Tell her you'd love to try again another time, if she'll let you. Whether she reaches orgasm or not, end your session by massaging her thighs and lower legs. Then wrap your hands around one arm and slide down to her fingertips. Repeat with the other arm. Massage her forehead and temples, run your fingers through her hair, and end with a warm, soft kiss and a thank you for such a delightful experience.

Turning the Massage Tables

Tonight, it's his turn to enjoy a "sexy spa" night. For this, you can follow the suggestions I gave him in the scenario above: Set up a "spa" appointment by telling him you'd like to spoil him with a sexy massage. As he did with you, have him shower or bathe and meet you in the bedroom. Get the room ready with candles, soft music, your massage oil or baby oil ready on the bedside table, and an old sheet or towels on the bed to protect the linens.

Get naked, slip on your bathrobe and wait for him to come out of the shower. From here, you can go through some variation of the routine outlined in my instructions for giving you a full-body massage. The only part that requires a little rewriting is the happy ending, should he desire one. Like you, he may enjoy a purely relaxing, non-sexual massage but, chances are, having your well-oiled hands rubbing and touching his entire body will eventually get him randy. If, after several minutes of body massage, you notice him sporting an erection, don't let it be the boss of you. Continue the massage as if nothing's happened. By not immediately attending to his erection, you will not only heighten his anticipation and arousal but force him to experience the sensations throughout his body—good exercise in being less genitally focused.

- -

Quick Tip:
Good Scents
Make sure the scent of any oils or candles is one you both like and isn't so overbearing that it leaves you both gasping, in a bad way.

- -

When you're ready to get naughty, let your bathrobe fall open and trail your breasts across his bum if he's on his stomach or briefly brush your nipples across his penis if he's on his back. If you have long hair, dangle it across his chest and all the way down his body. Intersperse this type of teasing with regular massage until you can feel him aching for you to touch him sexually. If he's not already on his back, gently turn him over. Straddle him, with your bum resting lightly on his upper thighs. Facing him in this position, run your well-oiled hands up and down his torso and across his chest. With your hands flat and fingers pointing outward on either side of his pelvis, slide your thumbs down into the crease where his thighs meet his groin. Press into the crease and slide your thumbs down, alongside his boys and across his perineum (the smooth stretch of skin between his boys and his bum), and back up again. Repeat. As his sexual excitement rises, you can decide what to do with it. You can "massage" him all the way to orgasm (for more instruction on this, see "Hand Job for Him" on page 100) or you may want to climb on board and enjoy the ride. Guaranteed, if he wasn't a fan of massages already, he will be now!

> **Intersperse this type of teasing with regular massage until you can feel him aching for you.**

- -

Quick Tip: Table It
The bed is the most common and obvious spot to perform a full-body massage. But if massage is something you both really enjoy and want to get more serious about, splurge on a massage table.

- -

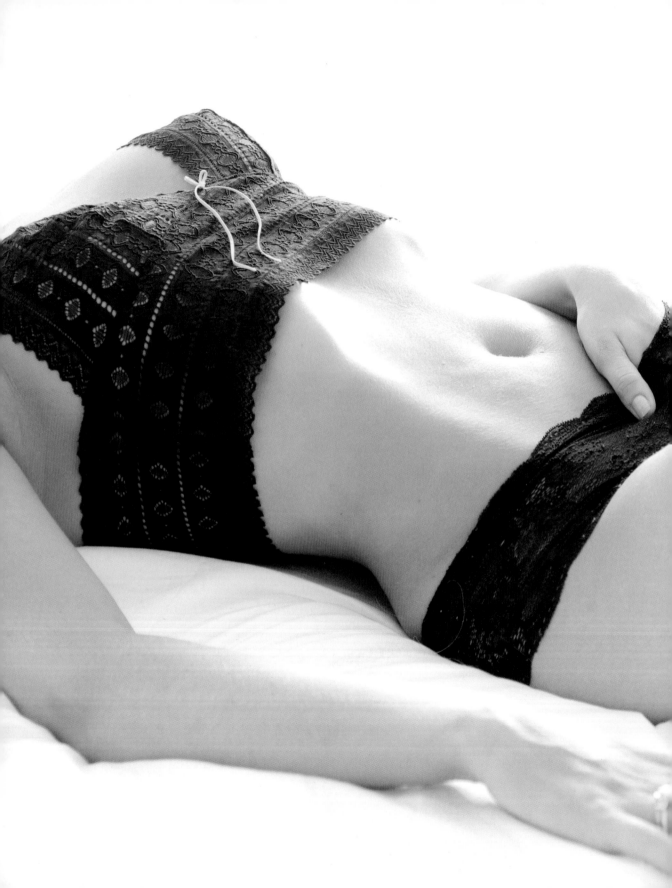

Chapter Seven
MASTURBATION

A section on self-pleasure may seem odd in a book about sex for couples, but the fact is that it's unrealistic to think your partner will be able to figure out how to please you if you haven't figured out for yourself what makes you purr. And the best way to figure that out is through self-exploration; in other words, by masturbating. It allows you to get to know your body and its sexual responses, how you like to be touched and what it takes to get you off. Also, when you're by yourself and no one is watching, chances are you'll be less inhibited and self-conscious, making masturbation a perfect opportunity to experiment and expand your sexual horizons. This, in turn, will keep your sex life together more interesting and exciting, because you'll both be able to bring new material to the table from time to time.

But despite its moniker, self-pleasure need not always be a solo activity. Masturbating for one another can be both a turn-on and a great teaching method. As they say, a picture is worth a thousand words. Mutual masturbation is also a real time saver if you're both wanting to get off in a hurry.

MASTURBATION FOR HER

While it's true that one of the best ways for him to find out how you like to be touched is to watch you masturbate, this advice is hardly helpful if you don't happen to have a lot of experience in this department. Unfortunately, while guys are pretty much expected to start masturbating as soon as puberty hits, we're less comfortable thinking that young women might engage in the same activity. As a result, many women grow up thinking that masturbation is inappropriate and are uncomfortable touching themselves or giving themselves pleasure. Which is a shame, given that masturbation is such an excellent way to get to know your own body and its sexual responses. So, whether you've been masturbating since you discovered the joys of a removable shower head as a teenager or are less experienced—maybe even uncomfortable—with the idea of self-pleasure, I highly encourage you to find the time for some self-love in your life.

And not just so you can show him what you like. Consider the other benefits of self-pleasure. Masturbation puts you in touch both literally and figuratively with your body. It eases tension, relieves menstrual cramps and releases mood-elevating hormones (see, he benefits here too!). It's a much more fun way to procrastinate than organizing the linen closet. And you're free to experiment without worrying about how you look, how you sound or if you've come "yet."

> 66 You'll be more inspired if you know you can literally take matters into your own hands at any time and finish the deed. 99

Moreover, as a master masturbator, if you have trouble reaching orgasm with your partner, it's just a matter of showing him how to get you there. Or chipping in to get yourself there, which can come in, uh, handy when you've only got a small window for sex and you'd really like to get off but it's not happening. Admit it, sometimes when you don't have a lot of time for intercourse, you know this means it probably won't result in an orgasm for you and you feel less motivated to go at it. You'll be more inspired if you know you can literally take matters into your own hands at any time and finish the deed. Because who's motivated to make time for sex if it's only going to leave you frustrated, right? So, be it a quickie or an entire afternoon affair complete with candles, satin sheets and you whispering sweet nothings in your own ear, take the time to figure out what gets you off. Just as having a good relationship starts with loving yourself, if you want a good sex life, you need to learn how to please yourself first.

TIME to PLAY

Five Minutes or Less

Come Quickly

Most people think that women take longer than men to orgasm. So you might find it hard to believe that, if you want to, you can bring yourself to orgasm in a couple of minutes, maybe even less if you use a vibrator. (If you don't own a vibrator, check out the "Toys" appendix for some advice on what to look for.) Using a vibrator, see how quickly you can make yourself come. Place it against your outer labia. Move up and down one side and switch to the other. Press it between your inner and outer labia and slide it up and down the crease. Press it against one side as you turn up the speed. Do the same to the other side. Circle your clitoris. Vary the speed as you do this, turning it up until you feel your excitement build, and then turning it down again if you don't want to come just yet.

If you're using a phallic-shaped vibrator, slip it inside, varying the speed as you thrust. Use the fingers of one hand to play with your clitoris as you use the other hand to slide the vibrator in and out. Instead of a vibrator, you can also use a dildo (a non-vibrating phallic-shaped toy) for penetration. If you want to get real fancy, slide a dildo or vibrator in your vagina with one hand and use a small vibrator (a bullet-or egg-shaped model is perfect for this) on your clitoris at the same time. Now pat your head and rub your tummy . . . just kidding.

> **❝**If you want a good sex life, you need to learn how to please yourself first.**❞**

One Hour or Less

Rubber Duckie, You're the One

A nice, relaxing candlelit bath provides a great multi-tasking opportunity. You get clean, you relax and you have yourself a great masturbation opportunity. The water offers built-in lubrication and you don't even have to get up for cleanup. Make sure you won't be disturbed for at least fifteen minutes, longer if you have the time. As you run the bath, pour yourself a glass of wine, dim the lights, grab a waterproof vibrator (there are lots on the market—you can

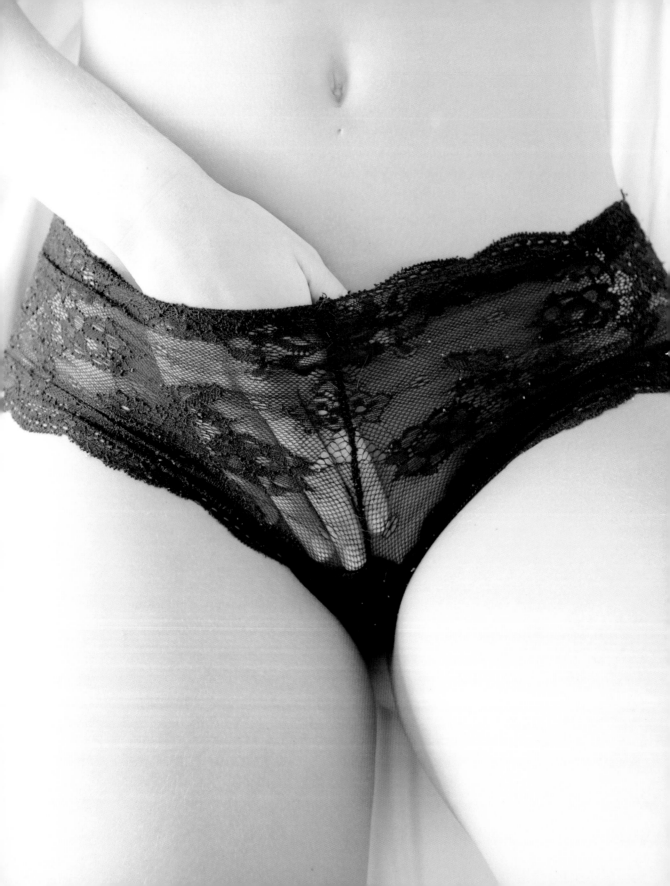

even buy one shaped like a rubber duckie!), then step into the water, lean back and get comfy. Turn on your vibe and slip it into the water, moving it around your breasts, up and down the inside of your thighs, and eventually settling it into your privates. Move it around to see what feels good — slide it up and down your outer labia, circle your clitoris, press it against the opening of your vagina. As your arousal builds, press the vibe more firmly against your clitoris, releasing the pressure or moving it away as you feel yourself approaching orgasm. Build up to orgasm again by holding the vibe firmly against your clitoris. Try circling your clit as you press against it. Repeat this pattern of building and releasing until you decide to tip yourself over the edge and feel the warm water mix with the lovely waves of orgasm.

AT YOUR FINGERTIPS

Bubble bath

Glass of wine

Waterproof vibrator and/or pulsating
shower head or Jacuzzi bathtub jets

Another way to enjoy the wonderful sensation of water during orgasm is to use a detachable pulsating shower head, if you have one. To do this, start with the head in spray mode and hold it over your clitoris to get used to the sensation. Switch it to pulse

mode and point the jet directly at your clitoris. Go back and forth from spray mode to pulse, moving the shower head around to see what feels good. Experiment with various jet settings to see what it takes to get you to the finish line. If you don't have a detachable shower head and you're flexible, scooch yourself under the faucet so the running water can rush against your clitoris. Or if you have a Jacuzzi tub, position yourself so that a jet hits your clitoris. Be careful not to jet water directly into your vagina; keep the stream focused on the clitoris. Oh, and be sure to lock the door. Nothing kills the mood like little Johnny walking in wondering what Mommy's doing to Mr. Rubber Duckie!

All Night

Spend Some Quality Time with Yourself

Ask your guy if he would do you a big favour and let you have a few hours to yourself. If you have kids, suggest he do something with them like hit the zoo or go to the park — you'll return the favour another day. Set a time for his return so that you won't be surprised if you're still, well, in the middle of something. Once you have the place to yourself, lock the door and avoid the temptation to clean, organize, do laundry, etc. Instead, use the opportunity to spend some quality time with yourself . . . in bed. You can get naked right away or leave on some clothing that you can sexily slip off later when you're more aroused. Have some lube or massage oil and one or more of your favourite sex toys at the ready so you don't have to get up for anything. Get comfortable. A tried-and-true position for most women is lying on your back with your legs spread, knees bent, feet flat on the bed, floor or closet if that's where you need to hide out to get some privacy.

AT YOUR FINGERTIPS

Lube or massage oil

Vibrator

Erotic movie or book

Read something erotic or, if you're comfortable with it, watch some pornography you like. These days, plenty of adult material is made to appeal to women. Go online and search "women's erotica" and "female-friendly porn" and you'll find some resources. If you live in a city that has a progressive sex shop, drop in and ask the staff for some recommendations. If you didn't have time to go shopping first, conjure up your own fantasy material. Think about him going down on you. Imagine yourself in a threesome. Whatever it takes to make you tingle. Once you're tingly and comfortable, you're ready to begin.

Let your hands awaken your senses by running them along your shoulders, your thighs, your breasts and anywhere else they feel like wandering. Pay attention to any areas that are more responsive and make a mental note to pass this information along to your partner later. Put a quarter-sized drop of lube or massage oil on your hand or squeeze it directly from the tube onto your vagina. Lay a flat hand over your entire vulva and lightly brush it up and down as you let your fingers explore its various parts. Slide your fingers between your inner and outer labia. Experiment with different strokes to see what feels good. Place the pads of your index and middle fingers together over your clitoral hood. Slide your fingers back and forth, up and down, and then in circles around your clitoris and see what you like. Run your index finger along the fold of one side of your inner labia, pressing against your clitoris as you slide your finger up and down. Do the same on the other side. Grasp your outer labia with your forefinger and thumb and slide up and down, squeezing your clitoris between your lips. As it begins to swell and become erect, squeeze the shaft of your clitoris between your thumb and forefinger and stroke it up and down as if you were stroking his penis. Run the well-lubed tip of your index finger along the underside of your clitoris from the bottom to the top.

> 66Every woman gets where she wants to go a different way. With practice, you'll find your own path to orgasm (and with even more practice, no doubt several alternate routes as well).99

Ultimately, masturbation technique, like handwriting, is unique to every woman. Experiment and pay attention to how each touch feels and how your body is responding. Vary the tempo and pressure of your strokes. Alternate long strokes along the entire length of your vulva with short flicks across your clitoris. Slide one or more fingers inside your vagina as you stroke your clitoris. As your arousal builds, use this private opportunity to practise a little dirty talk. Describe aloud what you're doing as you do it. Practise giving directions. Would you like your stroking to be harder? Softer? Faster? Would you like to feel your fingers inside of you? Imagine you're with your partner and vocalize what you'd like to have him doing to you sexually right now. Not only will this be a turn-on, you'll get used to hearing yourself say these things, which will ultimately make it easier to say them to your partner when you're together.

If you're close to orgasm but can't quite get there, focus on your breathing. Are you holding your breath? Breathing will allow the sexual energy to flow through your body. Inhale deeply and then slowly exhale, feeling the air leave your body from deep inside your chest. Continue breathing like this and gently rock your pelvis up and down as you focus your mind on the tingling sensations in that entire area. Check the tension in your body. Are you relaxed or are your shoulders up around your ears? Imagine your body going limp as you sink into the sensations. Every woman gets where she wants to go a different way. With practice, you'll find your own path to orgasm (and with even more practice, no doubt several alternate routes as well).

- -

Quick Tip: On Your Knees!

If you always masturbate lying on your back, it may be more difficult to come in a different position when you're with him. Kneel on all fours or lie on your stomach and imagine him taking you from behind while you reach between your legs and pleasure yourself. Or kneel upright, lean back on your heels in front of a mirror and show yourself how you like it.

- -

If you're close but can't quite find the exit ramp, try changing your breathing. Think of a really sexy image or scenario. Play with your breasts. Step up the stimulation. If you're penetrating yourself with your fingers or a vibrator, speed up your thrusting. If you're holding a vibrator against your clitoris, pulse it on and off. Slide it upward along the underside of your clitoris several times as if you're drawing the orgasm out the tip. When you start to feel the arousal build to the point where you think you might burst, stay the course and don't change what you're doing. If you don't get there this time, you will later. Be patient and don't give up. When you do finally come it may feel like your entire vagina just exploded or you may feel little more than a tremor. Don't worry, even practiced masturbators experience a variety of orgasms. With time and practice, so will you.

As you get more experienced and know what it takes to get you there, you can practise bringing yourself to the brink of orgasm, stopping for a second or two so you don't tip over, and then taking yourself back to the brink. The more times you bring yourself to the edge of orgasm and back again, the more intense your orgasm will be when you finally do come. If and when you do come, ease up but don't entirely stop stimulating yourself as you ride the orgasm wave. Continue providing light stimulation as you enjoy the delightful aftershocks of orgasm. Or, if you've got some extra time on your hands, take advantage of the fact that women don't need the recovery time men do in order to start the arousal process again and have another orgasm. Your clitoris will feel extra sensitive if you start immediately rubbing it. Squeeze some more lube on your hands, build your arousal and repeat . . . again, and again, and . . . uh, don't you have to be somewhere?

> 66 The more times you bring yourself to the edge of orgasm and back again, the more intense your orgasm will be when you finally do come. 99

- -

Quick Tip: Show Him How It's Done

Pick one thing you'd like to improve when it comes to touching her and ask if she'd be so kind as to give you a hands-on demonstration so you can learn from her technique.

- -

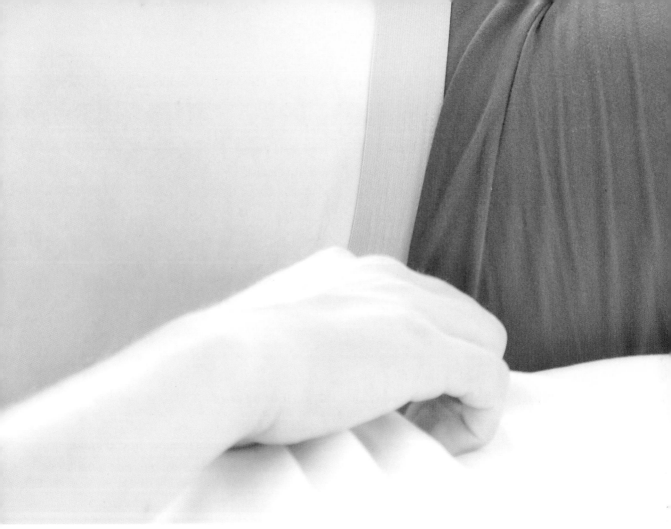

MASTURBATION FOR HIM

As I mentioned earlier, guys are pretty much *expected* to masturbate from a young age, so you get a much earlier start than a lot of women. As a result, you may have almost too much experience. What I mean is that, because you've been doing it for so long, masturbation has probably become routine and predictable. When's the last time you sprang a new move on yourself? You could probably stand to shake it up a little, am I right? Discovering new sensations through

masturbation is not just more fun for you, it also means you'll give a better response than "No, what you're doing feels good" the next time she asks if you'd like her to do anything special. Your sex life will benefit in other ways from some advanced masturbatory exploration. For example, has she ever complained that sometimes you're too goal-oriented during sex? That maybe you don't spend enough time enjoying the scenery en route to the final destination? You can use masturbation to train yourself to slow down and take some time to explore the surroundings.

And if not lasting long enough or lasting too long is an issue, masturbation can literally put you in better touch with your sexual response. You can use masturbation to improve ejaculatory control by making yourself more aware of each stage of arousal and learning to hold back before you reach your point of no return. If you have trouble coming, experimenting with masturbation can help you learn what it takes to tip you over the edge.

So instead of seeing it as a guilty pleasure to get over with as quickly as you can before someone catches you (a habit you might have carried over from your youth), use masturbation as an opportunity to explore your sexual potential. When you think about it that way, it's like you're doing her a favour too. Yeah, that's it.

TIME to PLAY

Five Minutes or Less
Make It a Quickie

Most guys have got this one down. As a young lad, you most likely learned to masturbate as quickly as possible so no one would walk in and catch you in the act. There's nothing wrong with that. As an adult, indulge in a guilt-free masturbatory quickie during your morning shower or wherever else you like to have a go at it. As with intercourse, sometimes a quickie is all you have time for, so relish it for what it is: a chance to relax, to release tension or to simply clear the pipes.

> **"**Use masturbation as an opportunity to explore your sexual potential. When you think about it that way, it's like you're doing her a favour too.**"**

One Hour or Less
Different Strokes

Set aside some private time when you know you won't be disturbed for at least a half hour, more if you can swing it. I want you to use this opportunity to break from your usual masturbation routine and experiment with some new moves. Start by creating atmosphere: Put on some relaxing music, fluff up a pillow or two, dim the lights, lie back and take the scenic route. Now, let's switch things up a little. For starters, that bottle of no-name lotion might have worked fine all these years, but a commercial lube or a quality scented massage oil (which won't dry up as quickly as lube) can add a sense of occasion as well as pleasure to your masturbation. Heck, why not go all-out and try some warming lube to shake things up? If you always use porn, masturbate without it and create a fantasy in your head instead. Or don't use fantasy at all and instead focus exclusively on your own body and the sensations you are creating. If you usually masturbate lying on your back, sit up or kneel facing a mirror and watch. If you always use the same stroke, try something different. Instead of fast strokes, slow down. Alternate between slow, light stroking and quick, firmer touch. For inspiration, take a peek at some of the fancy moves I suggest for her to use on you in the "Hand Job for Him" section on page 100.

Since no one's around to hear, by all means, make some noise. A lot of women tell me they wish their guy would be more vocal during sex. So use this opportunity to practise. Describe out loud what you like about having your penis stroked in a certain way. Talk dirty to yourself—it will make it easier to speak up when you're in bed with her.

> 66 Break from your usual routine and experiment with some new moves. 99

Extend your session as long as you can without letting yourself orgasm. Use the opportunity to practise ejaculatory control by bringing yourself to the brink of orgasm and learning to stop before you come. Here's how: As you get close to coming, pay attention to your breathing and the sensations you're feeling in your body. When you start to feel the urge to come, stop stroking for a few seconds to let the feeling subside. Circling your thumb and forefinger around the base of your scrotum and giving it a tug, or squeezing the tip of your penis right below the head may also help to stop you from coming. Experiment and see what works for you. With practice you'll be able to sense when you're close to the point of no return and eventually stop yourself from tipping over.

When you finally let yourself come, don't just focus on your penis. Feel the sensation wash through your entire body. Don't hold back. Moan, groan, scream, cry . . . let it all hang out. This will allow you to feel the kind of full-body orgasm she experiences when she comes. Who knows, afterward you may even ask yourself to cuddle.

All Night
Go on an Exciting Solo Adventure
You have a rare evening home alone; rather than switching on the TV, use this quality time to get a little sexually adventurous with yourself. Not only will this add some spice to your solo fun, you may learn a thing or two that you might like to

share with your lady. Once you're comfortable and have spent time getting yourself nicely aroused by lubing up and stroking your penis, experiment with some nipple play. Try pinching them gently or running a lubricated finger over and around them. Play with your testicles to see how you like them touched. (This will make it much easier to answer her when she asks, "How do you like to have your testicles touched, honey?") Do you like them tugged, tickled or squeezed?

AT YOUR FINGERTIPS

Lube

Vibrator or small butt plug

If you've ever been curious about anal penetration, this is the time to try it—when no one's judging and you're totally in control. Swirl a well-lubricated finger around the rim of your anus and see how it feels. If you're brave, slip it inside and slide your finger in and out as you stroke your penis. On the inside of the skin between your bum and the base of your scrotum lies your prostate—sometimes referred to as the male G spot. Curve your finger to reach it. Some guys swear that your finger back and forth across their prostate or applying pressure there at the moment of orgasm will intensify your pleasure. If this all goes well, you might want to graduate to a small butt plug. (Make sure it has a flared base so it doesn't get lost up there. Oh, it's happened. Ask any emerg doctor.) Apply some lube to it before slipping it inside. You can simply hold it there while you masturbate or gently slide it in and out.

Not quite ready for a butt plug? There are plenty of sex toys that don't have to go anywhere near your butt. Steal one of her vibrators (make sure you wash it with soap and water before you put it back!) or buy one of your own. If it's multi-speed, set it on the lowest setting and see how it feels against the base of your penis as you stroke. Move it around your scrotum, swirl it around the head of your penis or press it against the underside of the head. You may also want to get yourself a cyberskin penis sleeve, which you can lube and slide up and down over your penis. Test-drive a variety of sensations. Tickle your anus with a piece of silky fabric (preferably not your partner's expensive scarf) as you masturbate, or run an old comb (as in, one that is no longer being used!) across your testicles. The point of this exercise is to experience new sensations and to push you outside of your comfort zone so that you can bring this new-found sense of adventure to your sex life as a couple. The possibilities are only as limited as your imagination—and the things you can find around the house to experiment with that won't be missed.

MUTUAL MASTURBATION

Masturbation is generally thought of as a solo act, so mutual masturbation may seem like an oxymoron. But part of what makes masturbating together so intimate is the very fact that you're letting each other in on something that is usually private. You may both be surprised at what a turn-on it is to watch each other touch yourselves. And masturbating together is a great way to be sexual when intercourse feels like too much effort. Plus, I've already explained how masturbating in front of your partner is a fun and efficient way to show them how you like to be touched without having to say a word. Mutual masturbation has the same effect, only it's even more efficient because you're doing it at the same time. It's like cramming two lessons into one session.

TIME to PLAY

Five Minutes or Less

Who Comes First?

Lie on your backs side by side, set a timer and have a mutual masturbation contest. See who can reach orgasm first. If you feel self-conscious masturbating in front of each other, try closing your eyes so you can get into your happy place as if the other person weren't there, at least for now. As you both get more aroused, you'll start to relax. Sneak a few peeks over at your partner. If they're looking back, give them a smile to let them know you're enjoying yourself.

One Hour or Less

The Feeling Is Mutual

Mutual masturbation also includes masturbating each other at the same time. Essentially, this is like giving each other simultaneous hand jobs. You can do this lying on your backs side by side and reaching across to each other's genitals. Or, he can sit up against the wall or some pillows, legs out in front of him and spread slightly. You sit next to him, leaning back snuggled against his chest with your legs spread and stretched out in front of you or your knees bent, feet flat. From here, you can reach his bits from the side and he can reach around your waist to touch you.

You can also sit face to face on the bed with your legs wrapped around each other's bottoms. You can easily grab hold from this angle. He can certainly slide his entire hand, palm up, between your legs, though it is slightly more awkward to stimulate your clitoris from this angle. Certain moves that I describe in "Playbook B: Special Manoeuvres" on pages 94–96 such as "all thumbs" will work better for clitoral stimulation in this position. A phallic-shaped vibrator will reach spots his hand can't. Facing each other allows you to make eye contact, kiss and hug.

Once you're both in position and comfortable, use the advice I give you in Chapter Eight for how to give each other a hand job. As you both become more aroused, try to get in sync and match each other's rhythm. If one of you gets close to orgasm, slow down until the other catches up. If you can manage to make each other come at the same time it can be an incredibly powerful, hot experience. Don't be discouraged if this doesn't happen the first time or even if it never does. You can still have lots of fun practising. If one of you does come first, shift your focus to getting the other person off. Or, if they prefer, allow them to finish the job on their own while you caress their thighs, play with their nipples or simply tell them how scorching they look touching themselves right now.

All Night

Can't Keep Your Hands Off Each Other

Have a "hands only" date: No kissing allowed. Express your affection using your hands only. Hold hands on your way to dinner. Make a point of touching each other through the meal. Caress her face, rub his thigh, brush your hand through her hair. Cop a feel under the table. Give her a shoulder massage when you get home. End your date with some "hands only" sex. No intercourse, no oral sex. Instead, spend the entire time pleasuring each other using just your hands.

> ❝The point of this exercise is to experience new sensations and to push you outside of your comfort zone so that you can bring this new-found sense of adventure to your sex life as a couple.❞

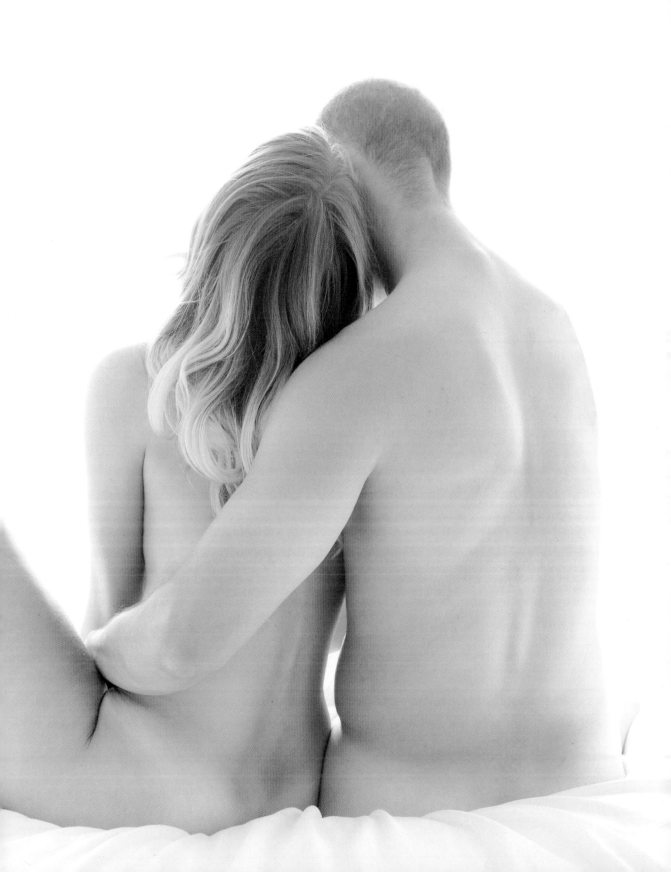

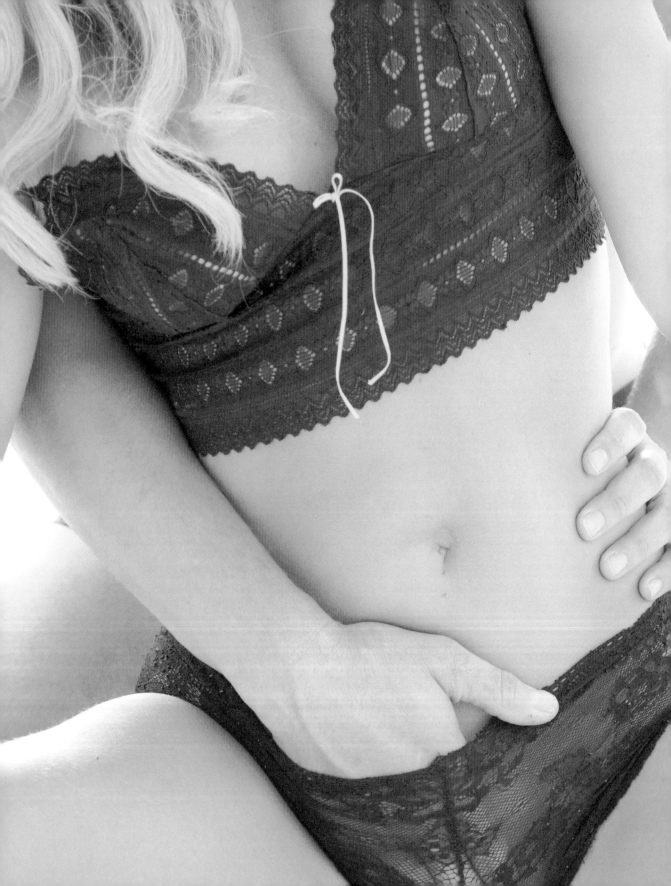

Chapter Eight
HANDS ON

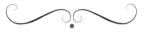

Now it's time to improve your skills when it comes to handling each other. Hand jobs can be as elaborate or as simple as you have time for. Once you both get really good at them, you'll be able to get each other off quickly and easily, which can be fun and convenient if, say, you don't have time for sex but you find yourself in a car together with a few extra minutes to spare before heading in to your friend's dinner party. If you've got an hour or, heck, all night, your hands can take your partner's privates to places their own hands haven't dreamed of exploring.

HAND JOB FOR HER

Getting her off using just your hands can be challenging. Does she like her clitoris rubbed back and forth or in circles? Does she like to feel your fingers inside her while you play with her clitoris? Oh, and what about the G spot? Where the heck is that, never mind the A, U and PS spots you've heard rumours of? It can be intimidating. Don't worry, I'm here for you. With some guidance and practice, you'll soon be playing her like a fiddle. Unless you don't know how to play a fiddle, in which case let's just say you'll know how to use your hands to make her experience pleasure beyond what she's ever felt before.

I tend to use the term "hand job" equally for men and women, even though it's more typically applied to men. I just can't get on board with the term "fingering." Not only does it sound crude and reminiscent of clueless teenage fumbling, it's inaccurate, as there is more involved than simply inserting your finger into her vagina. "Clitoral massage" or "vulva massage," both terms I've heard used, don't exactly roll off the tongue. Nor are they very sexy. "Genital stimulation"? Sounds like some kind of medical exam. So, for our purposes here, let's just call it a hand job, shall we?

While we're at it, let's debunk the myth that you can't give a woman a "quickie" hand job. I know that all the other books and magazine articles say that women take much longer to get off manually than men. Well, I'm going to let you in on a little secret: When it comes to manual stimulation, a woman can masturbate herself to orgasm just as fast as you can get yourself off. (If you're a woman reading this and don't agree or haven't experienced this, you might want to go back and read the "Masturbation for Her" section starting on page 58 while he finishes this up. Bonus, you'll not only learn to get yourself off, you'll be able to help him out if he gets stuck.) The more you practise, the better you'll get, and yes, one day, you'll be able to bring her to orgasm with your hands in less time than it takes for anyone back at the table to start wondering why you're both still in the bathroom. You don't want to make every hand job quite so efficient, but it would be nice to have that option, wouldn't it?

When you have more time, use it to hone your skills so you can turn your okay hand job into a "Wow, baby, you have magic hands and I can't wait to feel them on me again" hand job. A minute here, ten minutes there, an hour once in awhile, and soon you'll be a master of her domain.

The LAY of the LAND

For some men, the triangle between her legs might as well be the Bermuda Triangle for all its mystery. Get to know the lay of the land before you start exploring her, well, just what should we call it? It's not like the word "vagina" rolls off the tongue any more easily than "vulva," but for some reason, "vagina" has caught on as the catchall term for the lady bits when "vulva" is actually the proper name for the whole kit, at least all the stuff you see from the outside.

This includes the pubic hair (or lack thereof) and the mons pubis, a triangular cushion of fatty tissue on top of her pubic bone. This fatty tissue continues downward, culminating in the labia majora, the larger, fleshier lips on either side—her vulva's curtains, if you will. Push open her

"vulva drapes" and you'll see the smaller, thinner and hairless labia minora. A bit like sheers, these smaller lips block dirt and bacteria from entering the vestibule, the front hallway to her vaginal canal (where fingers, tongues, penises and dildos go in and babies come out) and urethra (where pee comes out). Besides protecting the inner bits, the labia minora continue all the way around her clitoris to form the clitoral hood. Gently push back the hood with your fingers and you'll reveal her clitoris. You'll see that it looks much like a mini version of your penis. Much like an uncircumcised penis, the tip is extra sensitive because it spends most of the time covered up. But check this

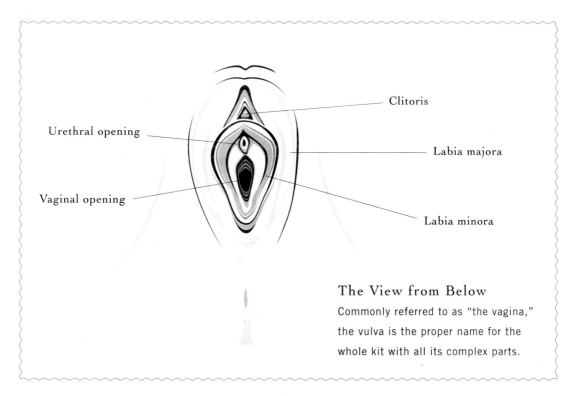

Clitoris

Urethral opening

Labia majora

Vaginal opening

Labia minora

The View from Below
Commonly referred to as "the vagina," the vulva is the proper name for the whole kit with all its complex parts.

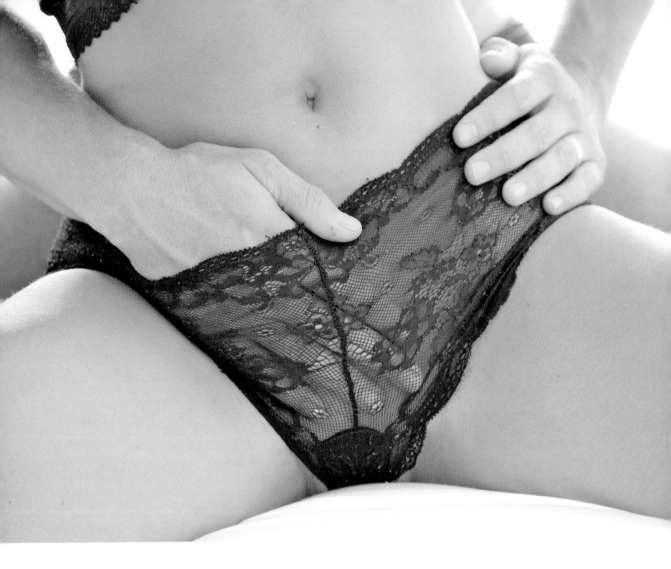

out: Unlike your penis, which has to share all the fun stuff with serious duties like peeing and delivering baby seed, the clitoris exists only for pleasure, containing six thousand to eight thousand nerve endings. How could you even think to deny this sweet little organ its sole purpose in life?

Don't let the clitoris's outward appearance fool you. It may look tiny, but this incredible organ extends back into her body and is actually the same size as the average male penis. If you pinch your fingers (gently!) just below the head of the clitoris, you can feel its neck or shaft. This shaft continues internally and splits off into a V made up of the crura, or clitoral legs, which extend up to five inches on either side of the urethra, inside the outer labia. The clitoral bulbs (yes, there's more!) run alongside the crura and fill with blood during arousal, causing the labia to swell. So, while the clitoral head often gets all the attention (and don't get me wrong, it deserves it), there's lots of yummy stuff going on under the surface in the surrounding regions.

Head south of the external clitoral shaft and you'll discover the aforementioned urethra. Keep going and you'll stumble into the vaginal opening. Enter and you'll find yourself inside the vaginal canal, the first third of which contains about 90 percent of the vagina's nerve endings. On the front inside wall of her vaginal canal just behind the urethral opening is the urethral sponge, also known as the G spot (more in a second).

At the very end of the vaginal canal is the cervix, which kind of feels like the tip of your nose, if the tip of your nose had an opening that dilated and allowed entry into your uterus, Fallopian tubes and ovaries. You needn't be concerned about that last bit here. For pleasure purposes, we'll be working with everything up to the cervix.

LEARNING the ALPHABET

You've probably heard of the G spot, because it's had a lot of press. But did you know that buried inside that lovely vagina of hers are also A, U and PS spots?

The G spot lies just inside the front wall of her vaginal opening—about a quarter of the way up to her belly button. The G spot got its name not because there is a button inside her vagina with a big flashing "G"

on it (though wouldn't that make things a whole lot easier?) but because a German doctor named Ernst Gräfenberg is often credited with "discovering" it. I could write a whole book on the controversy surrounding the existence of the G spot (thankfully, many other people already have) but suffice it to say that your partner can derive great pleasure from stimulation in this area, which is really a zone more than a single "spot." Given the right stimulation, pressure and alignment of the planets, some women experience G-spot orgasms complete with ejaculation. The liquid that is ejaculated is released from the glans and ducts surrounding the urethra. It's not pee, as some women (and men) may fear.

"G" isn't the only letter in the vagina alphabet. In recent years, the A, U and PS spots have been hogging some of the limelight. The A spot refers to the anterior fornix erogenous zone (rolls right off the tongue, doesn't it?). Apparently discovered by a physician in Malaysia back in the nineties, the A spot (sometimes referred to as the AFE zone) is also located on the front wall of the vagina, past the G spot, just before the opening of the cervix. Stimulation of this area—considered to be the female equivalent of the male prostate—is believed to release vaginal fluids and may just feel darn nice for her. Unless you have really long fingers, you may have difficulty

Spot On

Have fun exploring the alphabet, and discover new sources of pleasure for her.

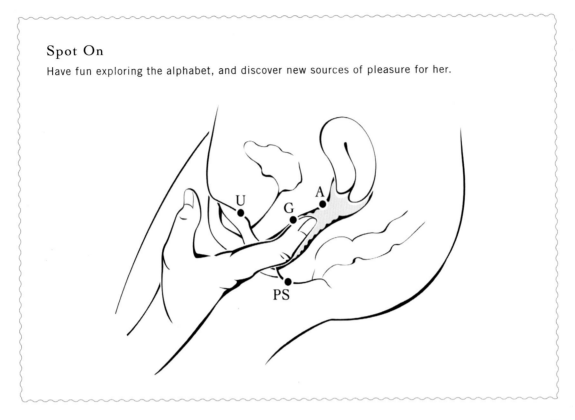

stimulating this area manually. Luckily, they now make special extra-long and thin AFE vibrators that are curved at the end to stimulate this area.

The U spot came to us via research out of the United States, and the "U" stands for urethra—yes, her peehole. Researchers discovered erectile tissue on either side of the urethral opening—located right below her clitoris—and thus was born the U spot. Using your fingers or a vibrator on this area may feel good for her. You won't know until you try.

P.S. Dear Josey, where is the PS spot? PS stands for perineal sponge (I know,

sexy, hey?). This PS lies on the inside wall of her perineum, the skin that stretches from the bottom of her vaginal opening to her bum. Much like her clitoris and your penis, this area of erectile tissue fills with blood and becomes engorged when she becomes sexually aroused.

If all these special zones, spots and areas make you feel you'll need to strap a miner's lamp to your fingers and start hauling maps into bed with you, rest easy. My goal in sharing them with you is only so that you know the lay of the land and can have some fun seeking new ways to give your gal pleasure. You're not a failure if you can't find her PS spot. And there is absolutely nothing wrong with either of you if she can't achieve a G-spot orgasm. Not all women can or want to. Simply have fun exploring the alphabet. Who knows, you may find she has some other spots no one's even discovered yet, and you can name one after you.

TIME to PLAY

Five Minutes or Less

Quick Tease

If you don't have time for a full hand job complete with orgasm, don't deprive her of the sexy touch of those lovely man hands. A quick dip can be refreshing and keep her wanting more. Pick a time when you simply can't take things further because she's scheduled to be somewhere at a certain time, like a work meeting or drinks with a friend. Once she's dressed, stop her before she leaves the bedroom, kiss her on the lips and tell her in your sexiest, sultriest voice to turn around and brace herself with her hands down against the dresser. Standing behind her, lift up her skirt or pull her pants down to her ankles, and ask her to spread her legs slightly. As she is leaning forward, slightly bent over, reach your hand between her legs, palm facing up. Outside her panties, slide your hand all the way back along her vulva, pressing your middle finger into her clitoris as you pass

over it. Repeat and count each stroke out loud. When you get to ten, stop and tell her to get dressed and head out or she'll be late for her appointment.

Bad Table Manners

When she's sitting beside you at dinner (at a restaurant with friends or at the in-laws', if you're feeling extra naughty), slip your hand discreetly under the table and lay it on her thigh. Run your fingertips along the inside of her thigh and then sweep the back of your hand between her legs before running your fingertips down the inside of the other thigh. Repeat as desired. This is even more fun if she's wearing a skirt with no panties. If she's a good girl and is wearing panties, slip your pinkie under the edge of the fabric and give her lovely pet a few strokes as you pass by.

Phone It In

When you've got a few minutes in the day, find somewhere quiet and private. Pick up the phone and dial your sweetie. Wherever she is, be it at her desk, on the train or in the middle of the grocery store, it doesn't matter because she needn't say a single word except hello. Then she can just listen while you spend thirty seconds telling her that you were just thinking about her and how you wish you were there right now so you could kneel down and slip your hands under her skirt, pull her panties aside and slide your wet, slippery fingers up and down her beautiful, sweet, delicious mmm, mmm, mmm . . . That's it. Tell her you love her, you hope she has a great rest of the day and you'll see her at home later. Buh-bye!

One Hour or Less

The Everything-but Touch

Ask her to schedule an hour one night (or morning or afternoon) this week with you for a special "body treatment." To build her anticipation, tell her to start thinking about what body parts she most loves you to touch and how she'd like you to touch them. When the time comes, set the mood with candles, music and a couple of glasses of wine, either in your bedroom or wherever you will both be most comfortable. Slowly undress her and yourself and have her lie back on the bed, sofa or rug. Tell her that no matter what, she is not to touch you. This is all about her.

AT YOUR FINGERTIPS

Candles

Wine

Lube or oil

After some gentle, warm kisses and a few sweet compliments about how stunningly beautiful she is, let your hands and fingers take over. Rather than heading straight for her breasts, let your fingers seek out the special places she likes to have touched. It might be behind her knees, her shoulder blades, the inside of her elbow, her tummy or just below her armpit on the side of her breast. Don't make these feel like pit stops en route to your final destination. Spend time at each one.

Quick Tip:
Colour Commentary

Communicate your enthusiasm and appreciation. When you're touching her, tell her what you like about it and describe what you see or what you're about to do. No need to give a play-by-play, but letting her know what you're about to do opens up the dialogue and may well encourage her to offer some useful input. More importantly, it tells her you're present and really happy to be there.

Take her breath away by lightly dragging your fingertips back and forth along the inside of her thigh. Be in the moment and put meaning and intention behind your touch. Pay attention to how her skin feels and get to know every inch of her body. Imagine tiny electric currents flowing between your fingertips and her skin. When you get to her breasts, gingerly trace your fingertips across the skin where her breasts gently slope from her chest and continue along the underside. Tell her to close her eyes and guess the words you're spelling across her breasts with your fingertips. Brush the underside of her breasts with your fingertips, and follow this with a gentle squeeze of her nipple, rolling lightly between your thumb and forefinger. Every few rolls, give it a gentle squeeze. Ask her to name which part of her breasts she would like you to touch and to give you instructions for how she'd like you to touch it. Example: Nipples—Circle slowly with fingertips ten times each. Dab some lube or saliva on your fingertips and grant her wish.

Quick Tip:
Periodically Sensitive
Some women's breasts are more tender right before their period and will need to be handled extra gently.

Move from her breasts to her shoulders, tummy, thighs, calves, the arch of her foot. Keep in mind that what you don't touch is as important as what you do. If you know that brushing your fingertips along the inside of her thigh makes her crazy, give the area one or two quick brushes, move on and revisit later. This is all part of the tease and it will drive her deliciously crazy. Work her entire body like this for as long as you've got, avoiding anything but the briefest brush with her sweetest spot. You may find that after half an hour or so, you both realize you actually have more time than you thought at first and want to take things further. I leave that up to you.

Bathing Beauty

Tell her with a twinkle in your eye that you'd like to draw her a bath and ask her to slip into her bathrobe and nothing else. Once this becomes a regular part of your sexual repertoire, she'll start to tingle as soon as she hears those words. Pull out the usual . . . candles, her favourite bubble bath and some nice soap and, if you have a detachable shower head, remove it from its bracket so you'll be able to reach it later. Pop open a bottle of wine if you like and slip into the tub. Sit back with your legs spread and invite her to join you in the sudsy water, with her resting her back against your chest so you can reach your arms around her. Let her sink into you and relax for a few minutes as she enjoys a few sips of wine and drinks in the romantic atmosphere.

AT YOUR FINGERTIPS

Her favourite bubble bath

Soap

Candles

Wine

Detachable pulsating shower head

(optional)

Take the soap and lather up her shoulders and breasts, caressing them with your slippery, soapy wet hands. Plant sweet kisses on her neck and shoulders. Grab the detachable shower head and ask her to turn on the tap. Get the water to just the right temperature and direct the shower spray onto her shoulders and neck, varying the pulsations. As she relaxes, move the shower head to her front, letting the spray hit her breasts. If her knees are slightly bent, you should be able to direct the spray toward her inner thighs. Move it down the inside of one thigh, let it pass briefly between her legs and then move it back up the inside of the other thigh. Do this again but on a more intense pulsation setting. Go back to the spray setting.

When you sense her becoming aroused, hold the shower head more directly between her legs. Be sure to aim the spray down so that it doesn't flow directly into her vagina. As you hold the head about an inch away from her clitoral hood with one hand, use the other hand to vary the pulsation setting. As she becomes more aroused, hold the more intense pulsation setting longer each time. When you feel her tense up and her hips thrust toward the shower head, she is nearing orgasm. Keep the pulsation steady at this point until she climaxes. If you don't have a pulsing shower head, you might want to invest in one. In the mean-

time, you can use your lovely slippery, wet hands to bring her to orgasm. For technical assistance, read through the "All Night" scenario on page 84.

Gee, That Feels Good

Using your hands to experiment with G-spot stimulation is great because fingers give you more detailed tactile feedback than a penis or a toy. But you can also use a G-spot vibrator or a dildo that has a curved shaft designed especially to hit her G spot. Before you invite her to embark on your G-spot expedition, delicately suggest that she empty her bladder first. The reason I say this is that, during G-spot stimulation, she may feel the need to push, and if she hasn't gone to the bathroom she may be concerned that pushing will make her wet the bed. You don't want her to worry her pretty little head about this so, to allow her to enjoy the evening's activities with wild abandon, suggest she pee first.

Niceties out of the way, let us begin. It should go without saying at this point that like any other hand job activity, an evening of G-spot exploration must begin with the usual warm-up—kissing, touching, etc. Using all your new-found hand job skills, you should soon have her sufficiently stoked for a journey to the G spot. If she isn't in position already, have her lie on her back and, palm facing up, slide a finger or two inside her vagina. Add a stimulating lube or gel to your finger when exploring her G spot. Applied to the this, or any other spot for that matter, these specialized formulas cause a tingling sensation. It's like bringing bubbly to a party: It makes the occasion more festive. Once inside, curve the tips of your fingers toward the front inside wall of her vagina and you should feel an almost ridged patch of skin, a bit like the bumpy roof of your mouth. Welcome to her G spot.

Quick Tip:
Alternate Route

He may not get you where you want to go exactly the same way you do on you own. Don't worry about it. His unique touch may help you discover a new route you've never taken before.

Slide the pads of your fingers back and forth across the entire area. You may feel it swell as you do this because the Skene's gland, which makes up the G spot, is filling with liquid. As you continue stimulation, she may start to feel like she wants to push and a pressure like she has to pee. But, smart fellow that you are, since you had her go beforehand, she can follow her vagina's instinct to bear down without worrying. Stimulate her clitoris using the index and middle fingers of your other hand, or by cir-

cling a small vibrator around it, as you continue to rub your fingers over her G spot. Continued stimulation of the G spot may cause her to ejaculate. Or it may not. That's okay too. It's still a fun letter to play with.

If you want to continue exploring the alphabet, the A and U spots are deeper in the vagina, so unless you have really long fingers, you have a better chance of hitting these with a toy or your penis. However, you can easily use your fingers to stimulate her PS spot. Slide one or two curved fingers, facing down, along the back inside wall of her vagina toward her behind. Or make a motion like you're hitchhiking. Place the flat of your thumb against the bottom of her vaginal opening. Curl your thumb as you slide it into her vagina and down along the back inside wall. Slide in and out and back and forth along her PS spot. You can also use a G-spot vibrator on her PS spot. Just flip it around so the curved tip hits the back inside wall of her vagina instead of the front, and alternate sliding it back and forth and in and out over the area. If you want to complete the picture, use your other hand or a vibrator against her clitoris (for more help with this, check out the "All Night" scenario on the next page) to bring her to orgasm. There, see? I knew you could. And see all that fun and pleasure you've given her and you haven't even officially had "sex" yet!

All Night

Handyman Special

Send her an email invitation for a One-way Pleasure Party. Administered by You. BYOSU (Bring Your Own Sexy Underwear). Location: Your Bedroom. Once she's arrived in her best undies, have her lie back on the bed and keep her sexy pants on for now. Start the festivities by serving up some hot kisses and several minutes of sexy body caressing. When she feels sufficiently welcomed by her host, start the main attraction. Slowly run your fingertip back and forth underneath the edges of her panties. Glide your fingertip lightly along the entire length of her loveliness through

---

Quick Tip:
Mix It Up

In general, the more turned on she is, the rougher and more intense your touch can be. A variety of rough and gentle handling will cover your bases and keep things excitingly unpredictable.

---

the fabric. Pull it aside and run the backside of your hand ever so lightly up and down against her. Slither a slinky piece of material (grab one of her camisoles from her underwear drawer) or a feather back and forth across her entire vulva. Grab the front of her underwear and pull it up so

that it gathers between her lovely lips and tug tightly so she feels the pressure of the cloth against her love button. Then slowly and seductively remove her panties. Don't dive right in: Dance your fingertips along her hipbones and lightly graze her pubic hair (or the pubic hair area if she's a clean-cut gal). Run your fingers gingerly along the crease where her thigh meets her crotch.

AT YOUR FINGERTIPS

Dildo

Vibrator

Lube

I know you see it in porn all the time (not that you've ever watched porn, right?), but resist the temptation to head straight for the clitoris and start rubbing it back and forth with one or two fingers. If she's not already extremely turned on, this move will be too intense too soon and is more likely to numb her than arouse her. Instead, squeeze a generous amount of lube onto your thumb and forefinger and gather her outer lips between them. Slide these fingers up and down in opposite directions so that all the yummy bits in between get a gentle massage. From here, there are any number of moves you can try. For ideas, see "Playbook B: Special Manoeuvres" on pages 94–96.

Use the extra time you have to expand

Quick Tip: Changing the Combination

Each woman comes with her own touch combination lock, so what might have worked with a past partner may not work with your current partner. Keep that in mind to avoid a "one move fits all" approach.

---

your hand job skills and turn your good hand job into an awesome hand job. The easiest way to do this is by adding penetration. In fact, as you've probably realized, trying to continue using your hands to stimulate her genitals during intercourse isn't exactly the easiest thing to pull off. At the same time, one of the most delicious feelings for her is to have her clitoris stroked while being penetrated simultaneously. And I don't necessarily mean with your penis. Luckily, you have other things besides your penis at your disposal, like fingers and dildos (if you don't own a dildo, check out the "Toys" appendix for some advice on what's available). Even still, combining clitoral stimulation and penetration requires some coordination, so make sure to set aside an evening now and again to have some fun practising.

As with any hand job, you want to spend lots of time kissing her and caressing other parts of her body to get her sufficiently fired up. Then, after some time spent on the clitoral stimulation techniques I've shown you up to now, she'll be ready for you to bring your fingers to the party.

When it comes to digital penetration (that's digital as in fingers, not electronics), here are three things to keep in mind:

• Even if she is very excited and wet, don't hesitate to add more lube.

• If you can comfortably insert two fingers instead of just one, you'll make more contact with the nerves at the opening of her vagina.

• Curving your fingertips slightly rather than inserting them straight will allow you to make more contact with the nerves in both the front and back inside walls of her vagina.

Now try this: While gliding the fingers of one hand back and forth across her clitoris, insert the middle and index fingers of the other hand, into her vagina. Either curl your fingers up and slide them along the front inside wall, or insert them face down and curl them to slide along the back inside wall, along the inside of her nerve-packed perineum (the area between the base of her vaginal opening and her bum). Once inside,

Quick Tip: Get Your Game On

If you're a video game player, employ some of the same skills during a hand job—using a multitude of quick movements, knowing when to suddenly change things up so you don't get killed, and staying the course to get to the finish line—and you're bound to end up a winner.

maintain contact as you slide in and out with one hand and continue to play with her outer bits with the other. If you want an extra smooth, velvety touch, wear a latex glove (you can buy them by the box at most drugstores) and use lube with it.

Quick Tip:
It's All in the Wrist

If you watch her masturbate, you'll notice her entire hand and wrist get in on the action. Moving your hand and wrist along with your fingers will make your movements more fluid and flexible.

As an alternative to your fingers, you can substitute a well-lubricated dildo. While you slide the dildo in and out, slide the flat of the thumb or finger of your other hand back and forth across her clitoris. Tickle the opening of her vagina with the dildo for a while before slowly, slowly sliding it inside. Follow a few long, slow thrusts in and out with a series of quick, fast thrusts. Quicken your thrusts as she gets close to orgasm and try to get a steady rhythm going between pushing with the dildo (or your fingers) and

rubbing her clit. Like I said, it takes some coordination, but that's why you've devoted an evening to the experience.

If you're looking for ideas to help you practise, "Playbook C: Let's Get Digital" on page 97 describes specific ways to incorporate penetration into your hand job.

Finally, don't leave her out of all the fun. Let her get her hands in there too by rubbing her clitoris while you penetrate her with your fingers, or inserting her finger together with yours so you can feel each other inside. She can also guide your hand with hers to show you the pressure, speed and type of stroke she likes. If she doesn't feel comfortable getting her hands in there with you, playing with her own breasts and nipples while you're getting her off with your hands will turn you both on.

Okay, you've had some practice incorporating penetration into your hand job. Now you're ready to add another tool to your "I give awesome hand jobs" arsenal: the vibrator. After all, so much manual labour can tucker a boy out. Nothing says you can't bring in some backup. Adding toys to the fun gives your hands a break and introduces a whole new set of sensations and added excitement for her. You can use vibrating toys against her clitoris and phallic-shaped vibrators for penetration.

A small vibrator that slips over your fingertip can be great to start with because you can manoeuvre it in much the way you would your finger, but, added bonus, it vibrates. A small, bullet-shaped vibrator is easy to use in and around her clitoris. You can also use the tip of a phallic-shaped vibe, moving it in circles or holding it directly against her clitoris. With a phallic-shaped vibrator, you can go from stimulating her clitoris with the side or tip to penetrating her with it. Whatever you use, avoid any vibration directly against her clitoris until she is very aroused because it may be too intense for her. Instead, move the vibrator in circles around her clitoris, move it back and forth across her clitoral hood or press it against the side. Using a vibrator with different speeds, swirl it around her clitoris and then pulse it from low speed to high directly against her clitoris, holding it on high speed a little longer each time to see how quickly you can bring her to orgasm. Try to break your own record. Pull out all the stops and circle a vibrator around her clitoris with one hand, settling in occasionally to hold it in one place as you thrust your fingers, a dildo or another vibrator into her vagina with the other.

Quick Tip:
Words of Praise

If something he's doing feels good, let him know. We're all suckers for praise, especially from our partner. As you become more confident expressing yourself, take it beyond the basic "That feels good" and add some details. What exactly feels good about what he's doing? How does it make you feel more connected to him? If he's looking at you and clearly enjoying what he's seeing, let him know that seeing the lust in his eyes turns you on too.

Most women can come relatively quickly with a vibrator against their clitoris, but that doesn't mean you have to let her. The beauty of a vibrator is that if you get her close to orgasm and then she loses it, it usually doesn't take as long to get her back to the brink again as it would with your hands. If she gets close, pull the vibrator away or move it aside so it's not directly against her clitoris. Tease the area with the vibrator and eventually go back to more direct stimulation with it until she is close to the edge again. Keep this up, going to the edge and back again, for as long as she can take it. Or until you finally decide to grant her sweet release.

66 Adding toys to the fun gives your hands a break and introduces a whole new set of sensations and added excitement for her. 99

While it's not necessary to bring her to orgasm every time you give her a hand job, it's worth your while to figure out how to get there. If she knows you can get her off manually, it will take a lot of the pressure out of sex for her and let her enjoy the ride. She'll be eager to have you back knowing that you know what you're doing down there.

To go over the edge, most women will need sustained direct clitoral stimulation. The more aroused she is, the more literally you can interpret the meaning of "direct." Some women find any direct clitoral stimulation too intense. If this is the case, stimulate her clitoris through the clitoral hood. The most important thing to remember is that once she's close to orgasm, for good-

ness' sake, keep doing whatever it is you're doing. If you change pace or stroke at the crucial moment when she's about to come, she may well lose it, putting you both back at square one. And that's the last thing you want after all the hard work, I mean, all the fun you've had to get here.

The trick (and yes, it can be tricky, but practice makes perfect) is to tap into the exact rhythm and pace that will send her over the edge. You want a stroke that you can speed up and also maintain consistently for about a minute. This may be sliding the pads of one or two fingers over her clitoris back and forth, up and down, in circles or any combination thereof. Or place the flat of your thumb against the base of her clitoris and stroke repeatedly upward along the underside and over the tip. Once you find a stroke that is comfortable and seems to be working, get into a rhythm with it, speeding up and adding more pressure as she gets closer to orgasm. It may help you to think about how you masturbate or what it takes to send you over the edge during a hand job. You want

---

Quick Tip: Hands On

Encourage her to show you how she uses a vibrator on herself. If she's shy or uncomfortable touching herself in front of you, gently place her hand where yours was and whisper sexily in her ear that her you'd really love her to show you how she likes it. Lay your hand over hers as she moves the vibrator to get a feel for the pressure, speed and technique she is using.

---

consistent, steady strokes that get faster as you approach orgasm. Focus on the connection and the energy flowing between the skin of your fingers and her clitoris as if they were almost fused together. Imagine that you're drawing the orgasm out of her and into your fingertips.

Quick Tip:
Hitting the Sweet Spot

A simple "Mmm" says "Keep doing what you're doing." If she lets out a sudden gasp or an "oh, yes," you've hit a particularly good spot. When you feel her butt and pelvic muscles tensing, as well as her legs and toes tightening and/or her hips lifting slightly off the bed, she's either got a charley horse or she's approaching orgasm.

As she gets close to orgasm it's especially important that you pay attention to her breathing and body language. In general a woman becomes still as she approaches orgasm: She's focusing and trying to avoid any sudden movements that will throw off your stroke. Her breathing may get quick and shallow (almost as if she's hyperventilating) or she may let out several deep, sharp exhales. (Remember as a kid how you used your breath to fog the window so you could draw pictures on it? A bit like that.) She may seem to have stopped breathing completely. Whatever her "about to come" breathing style, you'll notice it suddenly becomes steady.

Once you hit on the right rhythm, keep it going until you feel her nearing orgasm (like I said, short breaths, holding her breath, remaining very still, bucking her hips, grinding in your hand, cursing up a story—with practice, you'll get to know the specific signs that your gal's close). If you're using your fingers or a toy for penetration, speed up the thrusting even more until she (hopefully) reaches her peak. Once you get more experienced at knowing when she is about to come, you can intensify her orgasm by bringing her to the brink several times before you take her over the edge. When you know she is very close to orgasm, slow down your strokes for a few seconds—just long enough for her urge to orgasm to subside but not so long that it disappears completely and you have to start all over again. It can be tricky to find the window here, but don't let that stop you from having some fun trying. See how many times you can bring her to the brink of orgasm without tipping her over, using just your hands.

> 66 With practice, you'll get to know the specific signs that your gal's close. 99

If and when she does come, follow through. Her main orgasm will generally be followed by smaller waves of pleasure before it finally subsides. Ride these out with her — if your fingers are on her clitoris, keep them there until her orgasm eases off. Her clitoris will be extremely sensitive immediately after she comes, so stop any direct stroking and instead lazily circle her clitoral hood or cup your entire hand snugly over her entire vulva, feeling the final pulses of her orgasm. If your fingers (or a dildo) are inside of her, don't pull out suddenly. Stay inside of her until her orgasm aftershocks end and then slide your fingers or the dildo slowly in and out a few times before withdrawing. Once she's come down from her fabulous orgasm, give her a big smile and a deep meaningful kiss that communicates just how much you enjoyed yourself. Then congratulate yourself on a hand job well done.

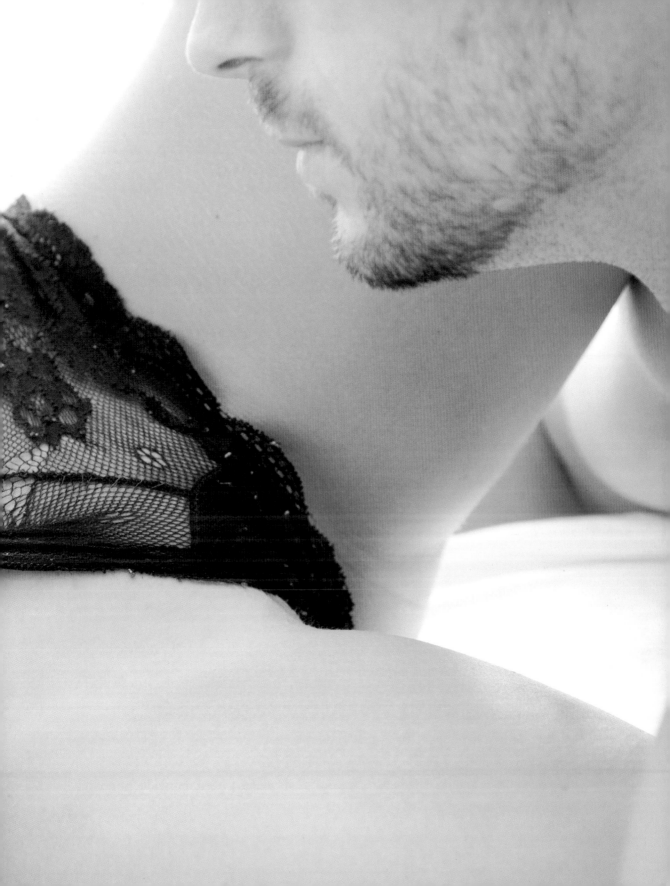

PLAYBOOK A
FIND YOUR POSITION

REACH FOR IT

Lie on your backs side by side. From this position, you can reach down to her genitals from the same angle she does when she plays this game by herself.

ON YOUR KNEES

Kneel facing each other on the bed with your bum resting on your heels. She can lean back on her hands and spread her knees to give you better access and a great view of what you're doing. In this position, you can use both hands to stimulate her genitals, one on her clitoris and outer genitals and the other for digital penetration. She can also lie back with her legs spread as you kneel between them with your bum resting on your heels. You can also sit between her legs with your legs (knees bent) straddled over her thighs, or lie on your tummy with your legs stretched out behind you.

> 66In this position, you can use both hands, one on her clitoris and the other for digital penetration.99

GRABBING A SPOONFUL

Both of you lie on your sides with her in front facing away from you, her bum nestled into your groin. From this angle, reach your hand over her hip (be sure to lie on the side that frees up your best hand) to access her genitals.

COMING FROM BEHIND

She sits with her legs bent open, knees resting on the floor. You sit in the same way snuggled in behind but with your legs stretched out on either side of her. She can lean back and feel your naked chest against her back and your penis against her bum while you reach your hands around to play with her.

BEDSIDE ASSISTANCE

She sits in a chair or lies back across the bed with her bum scooched right to the edge and her knees open and spread. Depending on the height of the chair or bed, you kneel (put a pillow under your knees) or sit cross-legged on the floor in front of her pelvis. From this position you can stimulate her clitoris with one hand and use the fingers of your other hand for penetration.

A FRESH ANGLE

She kneels and leans forward to support herself on her elbows or forearms as you sit behind her with your legs stretched out on either side of her. This position makes it easy to use both hands on her and introduces an angle and a whole new set of sensations she can't access when masturbating.

> **66**This position makes it easy to use both hands on her.**99**

GOING FOR A RIDE

You lie back on the bed and she kneels straddling your chest. In this position, stimulate her clitoris with your thumb. Once she is aroused, turn your entire hand on its side, fingers together, and place it between her labia, leaving your thumb cradled against her mons. Let her ride your hand, controlling the speed and pressure as she slides back and forth.

PLAYBOOK B
SPECIAL MANOEUVRES

THE SLIDE

Place the pad of your index finger (and middle finger, if you like) flat against the outside of her clitoral hood, pointing toward her feet. Slide your finger(s) down over her clitoris and then back up again, maintaining contact the entire time. Keep sliding up and down like this for a minute or so, being sure to keep things nice and wet. Vary this move by sliding your finger(s) up one side of the clitoral hood and back down the other, pressing inward toward her clitoris as you do.

THE V

Create a downward-pointing V with your index and middle fingers and place one finger on either side of her clitoral hood. Slide your V up and down, bringing your fingers together and squeezing her clitoris between them as you do.

SIDE-TO-SIDE SLIDE

Place the pads of your index and middle fingers flat against her clitoris and hood, pointing up toward her head. Apply gentle pressure and maintain contact as you slide both fingers smoothly from side to side across her clitoris.

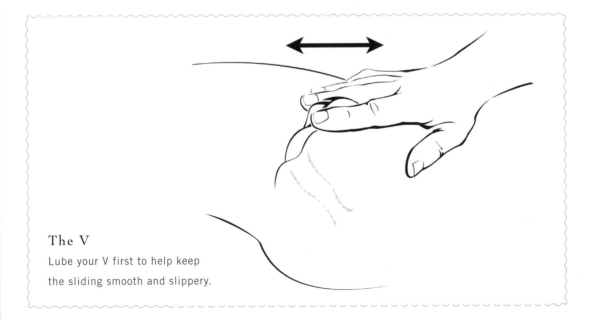

The V
Lube your V first to help keep
the sliding smooth and slippery.

THE CIRCLE JERK

Lay the flat of your index and middle fingers against the base of her clitoris and move them in slow, smooth circles, increasing the pressure as she becomes aroused. To practise, place your fingertips flat against your nose and gently roll them around the tip. Keeping your fingertips flat, slide them back and forth for a while and then go back to rolling. Now look around the bus to see how many people are staring at you while you're reading this and practising.

THE CURL

This move works best if you're lying or sitting beside her and reaching around. With your index finger pointed down, slide its flat tip down along the clitoral hood and all the way to the base of her clitoris. When you reach the base, curl the tip of your finger slightly so that it is lying flat against the entire length of the underside of her clitoris. Keeping it curled, slide your finger upward along the underside of the clitoral shaft. Repeat this upward stroke, keeping the movement rhythmic and smooth and your finger wet.

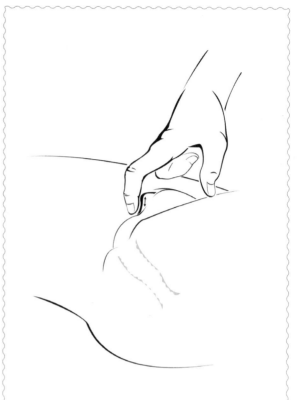

The Slide

The key here is to maintain contact as you slide and to keep the pressure firm but not too firm.

ALL THUMBS

With her lying on her back, kneel, sit or lie between her legs, resting both hands on either side of her pelvis, fingers spread, thumbs pointing toward her clitoris. Lay the flat of one thumb against the base of her clitoris and slide it upward along the underside of her clitoris all the way to the tip. Repeat this stroke with the other thumb and continue alternating thumbs for steady upward strokes along the underside of her clitoris.

THE PALM SLIDE

Sit behind her with your legs spread on either side of her while she lies back against your chest, and lay your hand, palm flat, fingers pointing downward, on top of her pubic bone. With your palm snug against her, start sliding down. As you pass over her clitoris, press the pad of your middle finger against the hood as you slide over it and continue down between her vaginal lips. Without lifting your hand or finger, slide back up, keeping your hand snug against her and sliding a flat middle finger in between her labia, then up along the underside of her clitoral shaft and back over the hood. Slide back and forth like this along the length of her vulva a few times, keeping the movement smooth and your hand and middle finger nice and wet. Try this same move with your palm turned sideways so that your index finger slides between her labia and up along the underside of her clitoris.

66Slide back and forth along the length of her vulva keeping the movement smooth.99

PLAYBOOK C
LET'S GET DIGITAL

THE DIP AND TWIST

As you play with her clitoris, slip your index and middle fingers inside, twisting them slowly as you slide in and out. Keep your fingers straight or curl them slightly while you're inside and swirl your fingertips around the inside circumference of her vaginal opening.

THE CIRCLE, SLIDE AND DIP

Circle her clitoral hood using the flat of your index or middle fingertip (whichever feels more comfortable). Every few rotations, switch and slide your fingertip up and down the hood and over the tip of her clitoris. Go back and forth between circles and slides. As she becomes more aroused, surprise her by continuing the slide all the way down to her vaginal opening and dipping a finger into her vagina (remember, focus on sliding along the front or back inside walls for maximum nerve impact). Dip in and out a few times and then, without lifting your finger, slide out and back up along her clitoris and over the hood. Circle, slide, dip. Repeat.

THE SQUEEZE AND SLIDE

Slide your curled index finger, pad facing upward, into her vagina and rest the thumb of the same hand flat over her clitoral hood. Gently squeeze your thumb and forefinger together so that you are applying pressure to both her clitoris and the front inside wall of her vagina. Slide your index finger in and out of her vagina at the same time as you slide the flat of your thumb up and down over her clitoris.

THE CAR WASH

Place the palm of your hand over her pubic mons with your fingers pointed up toward her belly button and the heel of your hand flat against her clitoris. Move your hand in circles as if you were washing a car, focusing on the contact between the heel of your hand and her clitoral hood. Switch directions. Once you've got a good rhythm going, slip one or two fingers of your other hand into her vagina and slide them in and out. Test your coordination to see how well you can buff her muffin while sliding your finger(s) in and out. Try this same move with the flat of your thumb instead of the heel of your hand as you penetrate her with the fingers of your other hand.

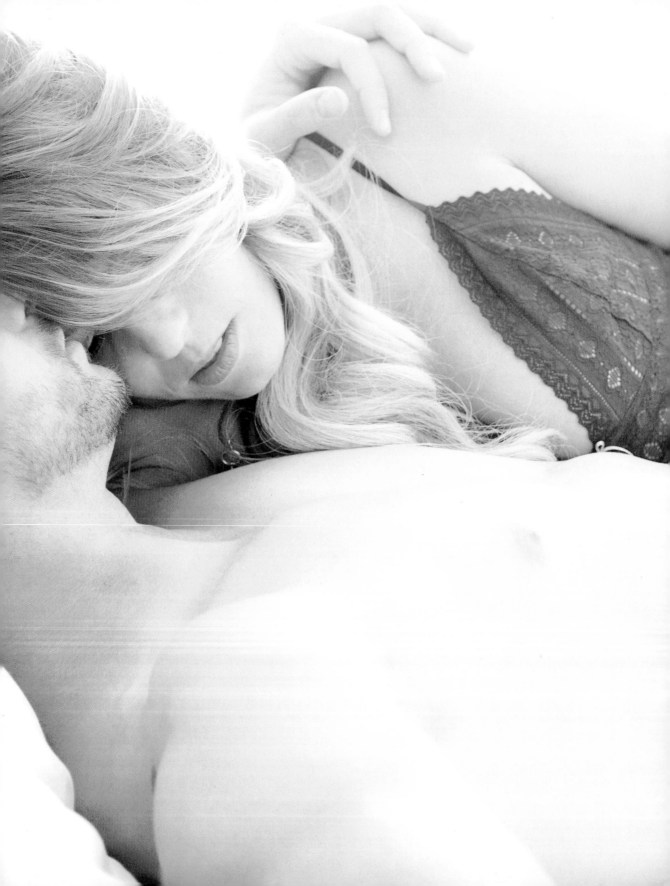

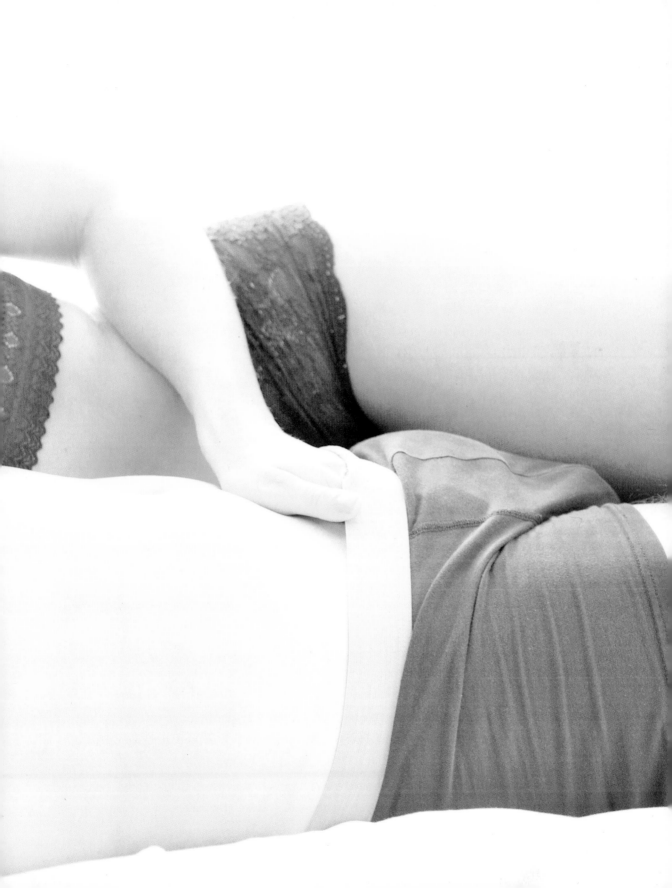

HAND JOB FOR HIM

Like I said, he's been at this since he was a teenager, so how can you possibly compete, right? Here's the thing: Getting a hand job from you is a wonderful and welcome change from getting one from, well, himself. He knows all his moves. With you, he gets the added thrill of not knowing exactly what your soft, warm hands are going to do next.

Hand jobs are handy, for lack of a better word, when you don't have much time. They can be discreet and don't require full nudity, which is convenient if you're time-strapped, too tired or not totally in the mood for sex and he's looking for some action. Should you find yourself with a few extra minutes when you can slip into a bathroom stall together or while you're going through the car wash, a quick hand job will tide him over until you both have more time to get intimate. The better you get at giving them, the less time they will take.

But honing your hand job skills isn't just about being able to get him off quickly. You also want to keep your hand jobs interesting. If they become too predictable, not only are you going to be less enthusiastic about giving them, he'll be (somewhat) less enthusiastic about receiving them. As I've said over and over, it's hard to feel motivated to make time for something you're not enthusiastic about. In fact, bringing lots of enthusiasm to the hand job is one of the easiest ways to turn up the heat. It's an absolute turn-on for him to see you completely enjoying yourself while you have him at your mercy.

There are lots of moves that will add variety, unpredictability and playfulness to a hand job. You don't need an entire evening or even a full hand job to try them. Take a minute to practise any time his penis is available: before intercourse, when he's about to get in the shower, while you're watching TV. As you experiment, you and his willy will get to know each other intimately. You'll learn what moves get him off quickly (for the times you have to dash off to your spin class) and what moves to pull out on those quiet evenings in when you have the time to lovingly torment him a nice long while.

The LAY of the LAND

Before you get your hands down there, you'll want to make sure you know your way around, so let's take a few moments for a quick anatomy lesson. Starting from the top (or bottom, if he's not erect), the tip or head of the penis is officially called the glans. It contains the urethral opening, or meatus, where pee, pre-ejaculate, and ejaculate, um, come out. The glans, including the corona (the raised ridge that sepa-

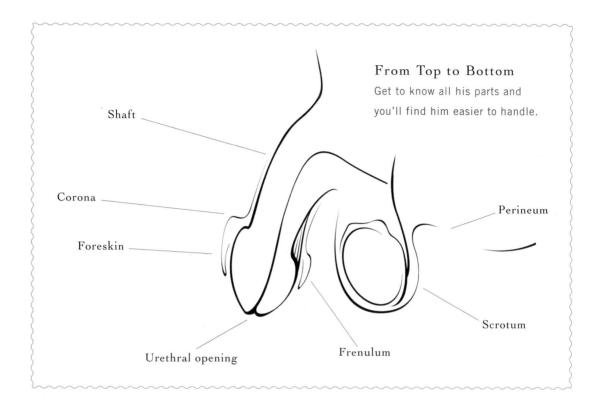

From Top to Bottom
Get to know all his parts and you'll find him easier to handle.

Shaft

Corona

Foreskin

Perineum

Scrotum

Urethral opening

Frenulum

rates the tip from the shaft) and the frenulum (the underside of the corona), is the most sensitive part of the penis. It's your clitoris's male counterpart.

Just as you have a hood over your clitoris to protect it, uncircumcised guys wear a hoodie over the entire head of their penis. This extra layer of skin is the foreskin or prepuce. Because North American women more often see the snipped variety, you might have been a little taken aback when you first encountered an uncircumcised penis and wondered if it came with its own manual. Actually, the original model has advantages. For example, without lube or lots of saliva, a hand job on a circumcised penis is a bit like going down a waterslide without the water. On the other hand, an intact foreskin acts like a tiny sleeve over his penis that you can slide up and down, creating its own built-in lubricating action. Once erect, both models look pretty much the same. Just keep in mind that the head of an uncircumcised penis hasn't spent its whole life rubbing against the inside of jeans or hanging out in the open air, so it can be extra sensitive.

The shaft is the least sensitive part. Despite terms like "boning" or "getting a boner," the penis is actually boneless. An erection is just a penis full of blood. That doesn't mean it doesn't hurt when you bend it, so be careful.

The scrotum, more commonly and oh-so-charmingly referred to as the "bag" or "ball sack," houses and protects the testes or testicles, his sperm storage tanks, pulling them up safe and warm when they're chilly and letting them hang down and get some air when they're warm, keeping his swimmers at just the right temperature to do their job. The line down the centre of his scrotum is not where he was sewn together; it's the raphe, and it indicates the internal wall of muscle that separates the boys. Between the scrotum and his bum lies the perineum, sometimes comically referred to as the "taint," as in "'taint his balls, 'taint his bum."

- -

Quick Tip:
It's a Wrap

If your guy is circumcised, mimic the feeling of foreskin by wrapping a piece of silky fabric around the head of his penis and sliding it up and down. Or use a lubricated rubber penis sleeve over the tip (see "Appendix A: Toys" at the back of the book).

- -

On the inside wall of the perineum lies his prostate gland, a walnut-sized juice factory that secretes liquid into his ejaculate so his sperm have something to swim in. Direct stimulation of the prostate—often described as the "male G spot"—via his bottom can be pleasurable. If he's shy about letting you inside to explore or you're not in the mood to go there, you can indirectly stimulate his prostate by rubbing, stroking or placing slight pressure on his perineum.

Now that you have a basic enough knowledge of what's going on down there to at least know your way around, let's get to the fun stuff.

TIME to PLAY

Five Minutes or Less
Have a Nice Day, Dear

When time is really tight and you don't even have enough for a full hand job, take five seconds in the morning to remind him of what he's missing. Before he leaves for work, give him a deep kiss goodbye as you run your flat hand up and down his penis through his pants for ten strokes, and then send him out the door. Sure, it might make his ride to work a little uncomfortable, but leaving him wanting more can be a powerful tease that will keep the idea of sex dancing in your heads, motivating you both to find the time to finish what you started. Keep the spark alive by texting him in the middle of the day to ask how he liked his goodbye kiss.

Race Against Time

While you're watching TV together (after the kids are in bed, of course), tell him you want to see if you can bring him to orgasm using just your hands during the next commercial break. Have some lube or oil handy so you don't waste precious time fetching it. When the commercial comes on, mute the TV, squeeze some lube into your hands and tell him to unzip. If he doesn't come by the end of the commercial break, stop and make him wait until the next one before you try again.

Morning Glory

Store some oil or lube in your nightstand and set your alarm five minutes earlier than usual. This will not only give you the extra time you need but will get you psyched for your early-morning activity. When the alarm goes off, give him a kiss and tell him to lie back for his morning wake-up call. Grab your lube and squeeze out a quarter-sized amount, rubbing it between your hands to warm it as you straddle him. You may find yourself greeted with a morning erection. Great. This will save you time. Glide your slippery hands up and down his penis, sliding them up and over the head and back down again. (For some fancy stroke ideas, consult "Playbook E: Tricky Moves" on pages 113–15.) If he wants to move to intercourse, whisper in his ear in your sexiest voice that you want to feel him come with your hands. If time is running out and you don't think you'll be able to bring him to orgasm, tell him how much you'd love to watch him finish the job. If you have long hair, tickle his nipples with it or scratch your fingernails along his thighs while you watch. As he's coming, kiss him deeply.

One Hour or Less

Causing a Sensation

You don't have to be the only thing doing the stroking. Encourage him to take a nice hot shower and wait for you on the bed . . . naked. While he's in the shower, spend the time looking around the house for things that might feel delicious dragged, slinked, tickled or slithered along his member. Once he's comfy on the bed, make your entrance carrying your box of goodies. Pepper him with kisses and caresses as you work your way down to his yummy bits. Start your sensory experiment organically. Let your hair dance over the head of his penis. Add visuals. Take your shirt off. Wet your finger with your mouth and trace it around your nipples. Look naughtily into his eyes while you caress your breasts.

Lower yourself over him and let your erect nipples graze along the shaft of his manliness. Then pull out your box of tricks and let the sensations begin. Slide a silk scarf along the entire length of his shaft.

Circle a string of beads snugly around the base and slide it up and down. Tickle the underside of the head with a feather. Watch him quiver with anticipation as he awaits each new sensation. Take the "hand" out of "hand job" and use other body parts to stimulate his penis. Take his erect member in your hand and swirl the head around your breasts and nipples as you stroke the shaft. Once you've driven him sufficiently crazy with a myriad of exciting sensations, you can decide whether you want to finish the job yourself or if you'd rather kiss and caress his nipples or stroke your breasts while he brings himself to orgasm with his own hands.

AT YOUR FINGERTIPS

Silk scarf

Feather

String of beads

Anything you've got lying around
the house that you think would feel
nice sliding across his genitals

Movie Buff

How about an X-rated movie night? Make a date to go see a film together. Try to avoid the opening night of a blockbuster when the theatre is more likely to be jammed full. Instead, pick a flop so the theatre will be mostly empty and you won't really care if you miss anything. Be sure to grab lots of napkins with your bag of popcorn and head to your seats. Sit in an empty row, preferably at the very back so no one's behind you. Once the lights go down and the movie starts, reach over and start rubbing the inside of his thigh. After several strokes, continue up, running the back of your hand across his crotch and down the inside of the other thigh. Come back the same way and repeat several times. Slip your fingers into the top of his pants (with the back of your hand against his stomach) and slide them back and forth along the length of his waistband. Go back to running your hand along his thighs and crotch. When you can feel his erection through his pants, look around to make sure no one's watching, slowly undo his belt buckle and unzip his pants. If you want to be really discreet, lay a coat over his lap.

Once you've released him from his trouser prison, wrap your hand around his penis and start stroking. Use some saliva on your hand to keep things wet (you could bring along a purse-sized bottle of lube, but he might not enjoy going out for a drink after the movie with his trousers full of sticky penis). With your hand circled around his penis, stroke up and down, sliding your hand over the head every few strokes. The fact that he has to stifle his moans and pretend he's deeply engrossed in the film instead of the delicious feel of your hand on his penis will only add to the excitement. Continue like this, quickening and steadying your stroke as he gets closer to orgasm. If you get it right, the movie won't be the only thing that climaxes. Use your napkins to wipe up and then enjoy the rest of your movie—if either of you can actually figure out what's going on, that is.

Rear Entry

As I mentioned in our short tour of the male genital anatomy, the male G spot is an area on the inside wall of his perineum. This is where his prostate gland lives. But let's leave the clinical stuff at the doctor's, shall we? What you need to know is that stimulating his G spot can be quite a treat for him. And if no one's ever gone rooting around down there, he may not even know it. Why not be the one to help him discover it? Of course, if you go poking around in there mid–hand job without any warning, he may not be too thrilled. Prepare him for it: Tell him you want to dedicate this hand job to his G spot. If he's wary, have him read through this section with you so he knows what he's in for. Tell him you'll be gentle and that if, at any time, he's not comfortable, you'll stop.

Ask him if he'd like to have a quick shower before you start, to help him feel more confident that things are squeaky clean. Then have him lie back on the bed while you smother him with kisses and caresses. Work your way down to his penis and spend time touching, stroking and petting it until he's standing well at attention. When he seems ready, start your journey with a little male G-spot massage. Keeping one hand full of his genius, use the fingertips of the other hand to tickle his perineum. Slide the heel of your hand across the area to increase the pressure. Lubricate your hand first to get the best gliding action.

If he finds this enjoyable, advance to some digital exploration. Make sure your nails are trimmed and filed. You may want to wear a latex glove or a finger cot (like a little latex sock for your finger), both of which can be purchased at most pharmacies. Whether you're covering up or not, use plenty of water-based lube (especially if you're using latex, which will be destroyed by anything oil-based). Ease your way by first massaging his bum cheeks. When he is relaxed and fired up, focus your attention on the immediate area of entry. Do not insert anything yet. Instead, use the flat tip of one or more fingers to circle and massage the area. Pay attention to his body language and feedback. If he tenses, go back to massaging his perineum. This might be enough for him. There doesn't have to be entry for him to enjoy anal stimulation. Massaging his bum and the area around his anus can feel great.

If he wants to go further, add more lube and lay the flat tip of your index finger (it will give you the best tactile feedback and the most control) against the opening. Slide the pad of your fingertip back and forth across it. Gently press against his back door and stop. This might be all he can handle for now, and that's fine. Check in regularly to make sure everything is okay and that he wants you to continue. If he gives you the thumbs-up, slowly and gently let your well-lubricated finger slip inside. Allow him to get used to the sensation. Once he is relaxed, it should feel almost as if he is drawing you in rather than you pushing in. To stimulate his G spot, slide your finger in past the first joint, curl the tip toward his front and slide it around until you feel an area that is slightly firm and bumpy. That's the magic spot. Now, using your best coordination skills, slide your fingertip from side to side, from back to front, or in circles across his G spot, pressing gently as you do, while your other hand continues to stroke his penis faster and faster until you feel his body tense, signalling his impending climax. Once he comes, let his orgasm subside before slowly and gently sliding your finger out of his bottom. You, my dear, have just given your sweetie a G-spot orgasm. Congrats!

All Night

A Proper Manhandling

You know how much you love tons of yummy teasing before he even gets his hands near you, so tonight, show him what all the fuss is about. Make him wait for it so that by the time you finally do get your hands down there, he's putty (well, okay, maybe putty that's been moulded into a really hard, quivering penis) in your hands. Create a warm, inviting, sexy setting, be it your bed or the living room rug. Light some candles and slip into something slinky to help get you into the mood. Let him know that this one's for him and all he needs to do is lie back and let you show him what you've got. Start with lots of sweet, soft kisses. Nibble his neck. Run your hands through his hair and give him your best "I'm about to rock your world" look.

AT YOUR FINGERTIPS

Vibrator

Lube

Slowly undo his shirt buttons or pull off his T-shirt so you can kiss and nibble his shoulders. Wet your fingers with your mouth or some lube and run circles around his nipples with them. Not all guys love to have their nipples played with. Gently squeeze and roll his nipple between your index finger and thumb and see how he reacts. If he jumps and pulls away, he obviously wants you to lighten up. Or he may discover that a wee bit of pain actually hurts so good. If he doesn't enjoy having you play with his nipples, you can still give him pleasure by running your hands across his chest and through his chest hair if he has any. Spend as much time above the belt as your imagination will let you. If he starts pleading for you to touch his poor, longing penis, tell him to—literally—keep his pants on.

> 66Spend as much time above the belt as your imagination will let you.99

When you finally head south, make him wait some more. Run your hands along the inside of his thighs and up along his crotch through the fabric of his pants. Hook your fingertip into the waist and graze the back of your fingernail along his stomach. When it seems like he might bust something, look him deep in the eyes while you slowly, slowly undo his belt and very (and I mean very) carefully unzip his pants. With his belt and zipper undone, keep teasing him by running your finger along the waistband of his underwear. Glide your hand sideways up and down the shaft of his penis through his underwear, then go back to sliding your

finger along the inside of his waistband. His penis will be absolutely aching to meet you by now (if it's not, your boy needs some more teasing). When the pleading look on his face starts to make you feel sorry for him, give him a sly smile and slowly pull off his pants and underwear. Drizzle some lube onto his penis and start stroking. Try the Twist, the Slide and Flip, or one of the other moves described in "Playbook E: Tricky Moves" on pages 113–15.

- -

Quick Tip:
Just Add Water
If things start to feel sticky and your hands aren't sliding smoothly across his skin, it's time for more lube. Some water-based lubes will come back to life if you add a little water. Ask if this is the case when you buy it. Otherwise, invest in a jar of lube with a pump. This makes it easy to relube without interrupting the flow.

- -

Of course, just because you've got your hands full doesn't mean you have to stop all the other great stuff you were doing before. As you stroke, give him a deep kiss, with tongue. With one hand on his member, use the other to squeeze his nipples. Scrape the fingernails of that other hand lightly from the inside calf of one leg all the way up his inner thigh and back down the inside of the other leg. Look into his eyes and give him a knowing smile that tells him how much fun you're having turning him on.

Once you've spent lots of time teasing and stroking his penis, see if he likes to play ball, or rather, to have you play with his balls. Every guy is different when it comes to how he likes to have his boys handled, and your guy may prefer you not handle them at all. If you've ever seen him take a blow down there, you understand why he may be wary of having you juggle his precious jewels. If he tenses up when you make a move for them, assure him you'll be gentle. Promise him that if he really doesn't like it you'll stop. In your capable hands, he may well discover that he enjoys having you handle his *cojones*. He'll enjoy this most if you continue to pay lots of attention to his penis, keeping him highly aroused, so get out those fabulously honed female multi-tasking skills. Use one hand to continue stroking his penis while you try out a few different moves: cup both testicles in the other hand and give them a few gentle squeezes; rest your fingertips underneath his boys and wiggle your fingertips; delicately scratch the underside of his testicles; wrap your thumb and forefinger firmly around the base of his entire scrotum and gently tug his balls down away from his body.

If you run out of ideas, or you want to watch how he handles himself, have him play with his own testicles. Be sure to make mental notes for next time!

Quick Tip:
Af-firm-ing Comments

When making specific requests, always be sure to phrase them in ways that are encouraging, positive and don't detract from the mood. For example, "Baby, I love it when you use a firmer grip on my penis" is more effective than "Baby, your hand feels like a wet noodle on my penis."

Like Barbies and Easy-Bake Ovens, sex toys are often thought of as strictly girls' playthings. But why should you get to have all the fun? Vibration feels good, especially against body parts that are full of nerve endings. It would be a shame for him to not experience the added buzz sex toys offer, unless your hands can vibrate. So bring some toys to your "play date" with your guy. You don't need a special vibrator for him: Any toy that vibrates will do. If you use one of your own vibrators, you'll have the added advantage of knowing how to operate the equipment and how that particular toy feels against delicate body parts. But just as you wouldn't turn a vibrator on and press it directly against your clitoris, you don't want to introduce him to this new sensation by simply pulling down his pants and forcing a vibe against the head of his penis.

> 66 Every guy is different when it comes to how he likes to have his boys handled. 99

Start by running a penis-shaped vibrator at its lowest speed along the length of his inner thighs. Slide the tip back and forth in the crease where his thigh meets his groin and then continue along the underside of his scrotum and across his perineum. You can do the same with a small bullet-shaped vibrator. If he's enjoying the feeling, run the shaft of the vibe up and down the shaft of his erect penis, avoiding the tip. Use your other hand to stimulate the head of his penis at the same time, circling it and sliding up and down, or using the Head Massage move described in "Playbook E: Tricky Moves" on page 115.

As he becomes more aroused, you can keep going when you move the vibrator up the shaft, sliding it over the tip and back down the other side of the shaft. If he flinches or gets jumpy, it may be too much stimulation for him, or the sensation may simply be unfamiliar and jarring. Men are so used to one type of stimulation, vibration may take some getting used to. Go back to

using it on other areas before trying again. Once he starts to enjoy vibration across the head of his penis, move the vibrator back and forth along the sensitive spot on the underside of the head. Hold it steady against this spot for a second or two, then go back to moving it back and forth. If you're accustomed to using a vibrator on yourself, treat the head of his penis as you would your clitoris and see what kind of reaction you get. Run the vibrator in circles around the entire head. Press the tip against the underside and hold it there for a few seconds. Continue pumping the shaft of his penis with your hand as you use the vibrator on the tip.

- -

Quick Tip:
Gentle Guidance

If he's shy about touching himself in front of you, tenderly place his hand over yours to let him know that you'd like him to guide you. This way, he can show you how firm a grasp he prefers or how fast or slow he wants to be stroked.

- -

If you want to take him all the way to orgasm using your hands, you'll need to eventually settle into a rhythm and pace with your stroking. Pay attention to changes in his breathing. As he gets close to orgasm it may quicken or deepen, or he may tend to hold his breath and stay very still so as not to lose the moment. If he's been enjoying watching the show up until now, he'll most likely close his eyes for this part. When his body tenses and his testicles tighten into his body, it's a good sign he's close.

Quick Tip:
Verbal Cues

If you want verbal direction, stick to questions like "Harder?" "Softer?" "Faster?" that require simple, one-word answers. If he's too far gone to speak, develop a code beforehand: One groan means yes, two means no.

Once you've got him here, zero in. Wrap your hand around his penis using a nice firm grip. If you've ever watched him masturbate, you've seen that he's not afraid to get a little rough. (If you haven't watched him masturbate, what are you waiting for? This is the quickest way to learn how he likes his stick handled.) Use firm, smooth, steady strokes up and down. Pay attention to his frenulum, the extra-sensitive area on the underside of the head of his penis. As you're pumping your hand up and down his penis, let the pad of your thumb slide over this area. Every few pumps, pause and slide your thumb back and forth over his frenu-lum. Use both hands and, as one pumps up and down the shaft, gently squeeze the head of his penis with the thumb and fore-finger of your other hand. Slide them up and down the tip so that your thumb glides over the underside of the head. As you feel him getting close to orgasm, ramp up the intensity of your strokes. Keep the rhythm steady, increasing the speed the more his body tenses up and the closer he gets to orgasm.

But you don't want the night to end yet, do you? Why not torture him a little, in a nice way, of course? Delaying his orgasm will intensify it and make him a very happy boy. To do this, slow down just as he is about to reach orgasm and let his urge to climax for a few seconds. Then, take your stroking back up and bring him back to the brink. Repeat the pattern several times. This is called "edging."

> 66 Why not torture him a little, in a nice way, of course? Delaying his orgasm will intensify it. 99

Keep in mind that most guys have a point of no return—that is, a point when no matter what you do, a freight train wouldn't be able to stop him from coming.

If you're trying to delay his orgasm and he reaches his point of no return, don't sweat it. There's always next time. If, however, you'd like to offer a little added incentive, tell him he has to cook dinner for a week if he comes before you let him. See how many times you can take him to the edge and back before you drive him completely out of his mind, and finally release him into orgasmic bliss.

Once he comes, slow down your strokes, avoiding the sensitive tip and frenulum altogether. Keep holding his penis so he continues to feel the warmth of your touch as the waves of his orgasm let up. When he comes back down to earth, slowly release him from your grip. If you were using anal play and he comes with your finger still in his bum, resist the temptation to pull out immediately. Let his orgasm subside and then slowly ease your finger out. Smile and enjoy the appreciative, dopey grin on his face as you grab some tissues to soak up the other sign of his appreciation.

Quick Tip: Body Talk

If your guy's not a big talker, pay attention to his body language. If he's shifting his body, you may be slightly off-base or doing something that's uncomfortable. If his body is very still and tensing up, his breathing deepens and he lets out a few deep, heartfelt moans or growls, you're on to something. If his breath catches or he lets out a moan, you know you've hit a sweet spot. Take note and give it some extra attention.

❝See how many times you can take him to the edge and finally release him into orgasmic bliss.❞

PLAYBOOK D
STRATEGIC POSITIONING

ALL THINGS ASTRIDE

He lies on his back with his legs together. You straddle his hips, facing forward with your knees resting on either side of him. This position enables you to use both hands on his penis and gives him a great visual of your upper body and face. You can also press your groin (either naked or clothed) up against the base of his penis to get a little action yourself.

HERE'S LOOKING AT YOU

He lies on his back or sits on a chair with his legs spread. You kneel between his legs, resting your bum on your heels if you're on the bed, or kneel on a pillow on the floor if he's in a chair. In this position, you can operate his penis with one hand while tickling his testicles or perusing his perineum with the other. He gets a great bird's-eye view of what you're up to and you can make sexy eye contact.

BESIDE HIMSELF

He lies on his back and you lie next to him on your side. You reach across his pelvis to his penis (make sure to lie on the side that lets you use your dominant hand). Circle the shaft with one hand (with the back of your hand facing his stomach) and use your other hand to tickle his testicles or play with his nipples, thighs or any other body parts you can access. He can prop his head up on a pillow for a better view.

I'M RIGHT BEHIND YOU

Stand behind him (perfect for the shower!) or kneel together on the bed so you're snuggled up against his backside. Reach around to access his penis. In this position, you can grab it from the same angle as when he masturbates. Only he can't kiss and nibble his own back, shoulders and neck when going solo. Nor can he feel your hot body pressed up against his backside as you breathe sexy sweet nothings into his ear.

PLAYBOOK E
TRICKY MOVES

Note: Use lube for best results.

THE BASIC PUMP

The old up-and-down pumping action is a perfectly good hand job stroke, especially further along when he's getting close to orgasm and speed and consistency take precedence over fancy manoeuvres. Wrap your left hand (or your right hand if you're left-handed) around the base of his penis to keep it stable while you circle the shaft and stroke up and down with your right hand. Grip it firmly, but not too firmly—you don't want to strangle the poor thing.

THE LADY PUMP

This is a more delicate, ahem, ladylike version of the basic pump. Rather than sliding your entire hand up and down his erect penis, use just your thumb and index finger (imagine the queen delicately holding a cup of tea). Start at the tip, gently squeezing the head between your thumb and index finger, and glide the pad of your thumb directly over the sensitive underside of the head—the frenulum—as you slide your finger and thumb like this all the way down and back up his shaft. Repeat.

DOUBLE FISTING

As in the basic pump above, circle one hand snugly around the top half of his penis and slide it down all the way to the base. Before the head of his penis emerges from your fist, circle the fist of your second hand and follow the first, so that his penis "penetrates" one fist after the other. Continue sliding both hands one after the other down the entire shaft in one continuous motion so it feels as if he is penetrating a nice, deep hand vagina.

THE O

Make an O with your index finger and thumb (as if you're making an "okay" sign). Tighten your finger O and place it over the tip of his penis. Veeery slowly squeeze the O over the tip and all the way down the shaft. Or just slide it up and down the tip, letting him enjoy "entering" the nice, tight, wet opening you've created.

DOUBLE O

Circle the thumb and forefinger of each hand to create two Os. Swirl both Os around the shaft of his penis in opposite directions, one hand after the other, from the base to the tip.

MAKE PEACE

Bring out your inner hippie and make a peace sign with your index and middle fingers. Gently wedge the base of his penis into the web at the base of your finger V. Slide your peace sign up and down the shaft, gently squeezing your V together as you slide over the tip of his penis, where he is most sensitive. Every few strokes, twist your V from side to side as you slide up and down the shaft.

THE TWIST

Wrap one hand firmly around the base of his penis with the back of your thumb facing you. Wrap the other hand upside down around the head, so that the back of this hand is facing you (imagine wringing out a towel with both hands). Squeezing gently, twist your hands in opposite directions around his penis, moving each hand up and down as you twist. Keep both hands in motion and the movements steady, slow and purposeful.

LET US PRAY

Press your well-lubricated hands together, as if in prayer. (What? You don't lube your hands to pray?) Then slide your closed hands up and down the shaft of his penis. This might freak him out if he's religious, but you'll know that much better than I. For a variation on this move, in keeping with the church theme (sorry, Mom), place your palms together and interweave your fingers as if you're playing "Here is the church, here is the steeple . . ." Place the shaft of his penis snugly between the palms of your hands inside the little finger cage you've created and simply slide up and down.

THE SLIDE AND FLIP

Circle the shaft of his penis so the back of your hand is facing his stomach (that is, if his penis is pointing skyward, which I suspect it probably is at this point). Circle your other hand snugly around the base of his penis to give you more control and keep him fully at attention. Squeezing gently, slide the first hand up over the head of his penis, then flip this hand upside down so that the thumb and forefinger are on the bottom and slide it back down over the head and down the shaft. Then slide back up the head, flip and slide down and back up, flip, slide, etc. Keep the movement fluid so it feels like your hand barely leaves his penis when you flip it over to slide back down.

THE FINGER SWIRL

As you grasp the shaft of his penis with one well-lubed hand and stroke up and down, lube up the index finger of your other hand, curl the tip slightly and swirl it around the tip of his penis much in the same way you might twirl your finger around a lock of your own hair. On the upward stroke, pause, keeping the palm of your hand wrapped snugly around the head of his penis, and twirl your finger around the tip as it's nestled in your warm, wet hand. This will feel a bit like he's inside your vagina, if your vagina had a finger that twirled around the tip of his penis while he was inside you. After a few swirls, slide your first hand back down and do it all over again.

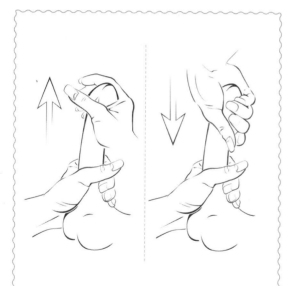

The Slide and Flip

During this manoeuvre, keep your hands well lubed and snug around his penis and the motion fluid.

THE HEAD MASSAGE

Give the most sensitive area of his penis a gentle massage. With one hand firmly gripping the shaft, form a "claw" with the fingers of your other hand: Bring your fingers and thumb together, place them over the tip of his penis, and slide them down just below the tip. Position your thumb so that it slides over the underside of the head where he is most sensitive. Slide your "claw" back up to the tip and right back down again without lifting off his penis, creating a smooth, continuous move. Keep up this head massage for several strokes.

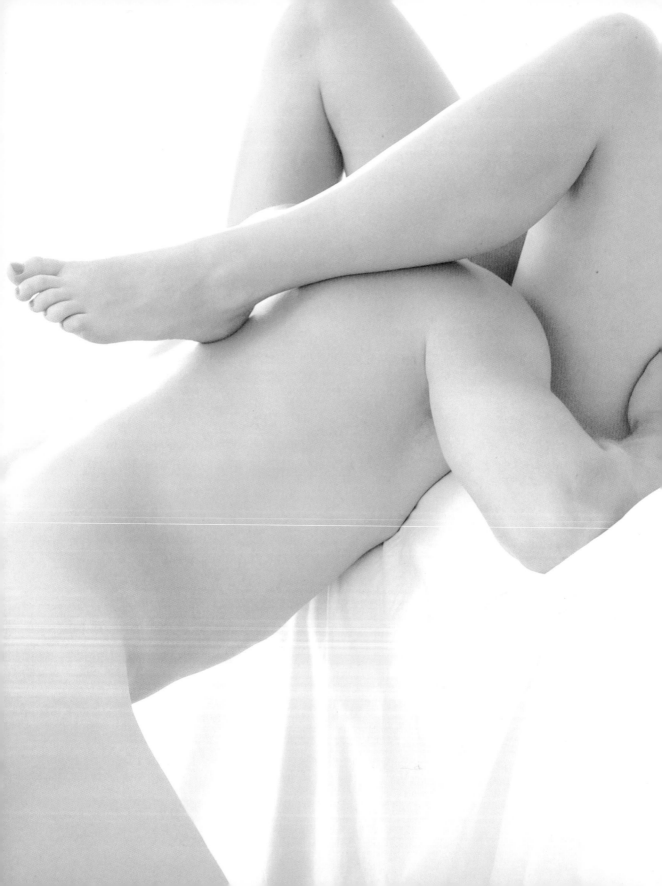

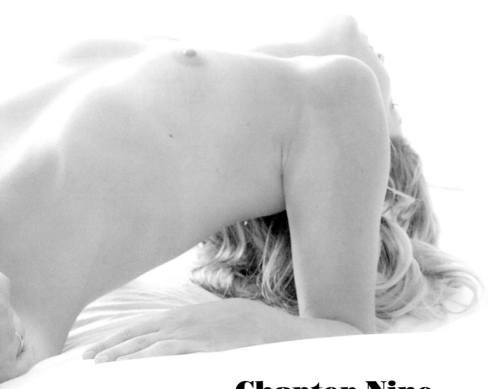

Chapter Nine
ORAL

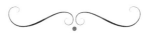

Feeling your partner's warm, wet mouth on the most delicate part of your body is incredibly intimate. In fact, some people consider oral sex to be even more personal than intercourse. There is something incredibly intoxicating about literally tasting your partner and about them making themselves so vulnerable to you in this way. Then there's the fact that it just feels pretty damn good, no doubt for much the same reason kissing feels great: Mouths are luscious, moist and soft. And slippery tongues can flick, lick and swirl into nooks and crannies in ways that fingers, hands and penises can't.

Like most sexual activities, oral sex can be adjusted to suit any schedule: Teasing her with your mouth for a minute or two moments before you go out can put some added sparkle into your evening, a quick morning blow job will make his day, and an entire evening devoted to exploring new ways to please each other with your mouths is the ultimate oral expression.

CUNNILINGUS

Do you want to know a great way to motivate her to make more time for sex? Get really good at going down on her. I know there's probably nothing you enjoy more than having your mouth full of your lady's lady bits, but she'll enjoy it more often if you learn to perfect your oral skills. I know it can be challenging, what with everything going on down there and the fact that your tongue doesn't come with batteries. But I can help.

For starters, learn how your tongue feels to her. Point your tongue and lick the web between your index finger and thumb. Practise short, fast, firm flicks vs. long, slow pointed ones. Swirl the tip of your tongue around your fingertip (imagining it's her clitoris)—fast and firm and then soft and slow. Notice the difference. Continue practising—varying the pressure and length of your licks, switching from a pointy, firm

tongue to a soft, flat one—until you have a pretty good idea what your tongue is capable of.

Next, don't avoid oral sex just because you're worried you won't have enough time or stamina to get her all the way to orgasm. A minute or two of oral pleasure here and there, possibly without orgasm, is better than none at all. And consider this: Many women who don't climax through intercourse can come through oral sex. If you don't have a lot of time for sex and you'd like her to come, you'd be wise to spend a chunk of that time pleasing her with your mouth.

Finally, anytime you go down on her, let her know how much you enjoy it. Tell her how much you're looking forward to tasting her as you brush your lips across her ear. Wet your finger and run it around the lips of her mouth and tell her that you can't wait to feel the wetness of her other lips against your own warm mouth. It may make you feel self-conscious and even silly to say things like this, but remember that words are intimacy for women. Why do you think she loves to talk to her girlfriends so much? If you can't speak up, communicate in other ways: Look into her eyes and smile gently. This tells her you're happy to be there and you like what you see without speaking a single word. A soft moan in her ear says "I want you and you turn me on."

Basically, you want her to feel like you've just sat down to an all-you-can-eat buffet and plan to get your money's worth.

> 66 Communicate in other ways. A soft moan in her ear says 'I want you and you turn me on.' 99

What's that? You in the back. You say she doesn't like oral sex? Right, I've heard that about some women. Listen, I wish I could offer you a magic solution to this problem. But if after you've done all you can to let her know how much you enjoy it and her, and tried your best to show her how good it can feel, ultimately, if she doesn't like oral sex, she doesn't like it. Pressuring her will only create resentment, so respect her feelings and find other fun things to enjoy.

TIME to PLAY

Five Minutes or Less
Aural Sex
She's always telling you she'd like you to be more verbally expressive. Here's your chance. The next time you find yourself alone in the car or at home while everyone is out, record a voice memo on your phone or, if you're set up for it, record an mp3 file on your computer. In your sexiest, most sincere voice, spend a couple of minutes describing in candid detail how you're going to use your soft, wet tongue on her most precious parts the next time you get a chance. Just as you would spend time warming her up in real life, do the same in the recording. Create buildup. Set the scene. Where is she? How does she look? What parts of her body do you kiss first? How do you kiss them? Softly? Hungrily? Tell her how much her sweet smell turns you on.

As you get more into it, paint the picture as you go. Use lots of descriptive words and compliments. Don't be too cheesy or cutesy (talk of "honey pots" and "Mr. Tongue" is best avoided) or too crude (think titillating, not trashy). Tell her how much you love going down on her and why. Describe how beautiful and sexy she looks as she gets more and more turned on and you bring her to orgasm with your mouth. Once you are satisfied with your work (and think she will be too), leave the recorder in her bedside drawer or tuck the mp3 file away on the computer so no one else will find it. Write her a note or send her a message to let her know that there is a sexy surprise waiting for her (wherever you left it) the next time she has a few minutes alone.

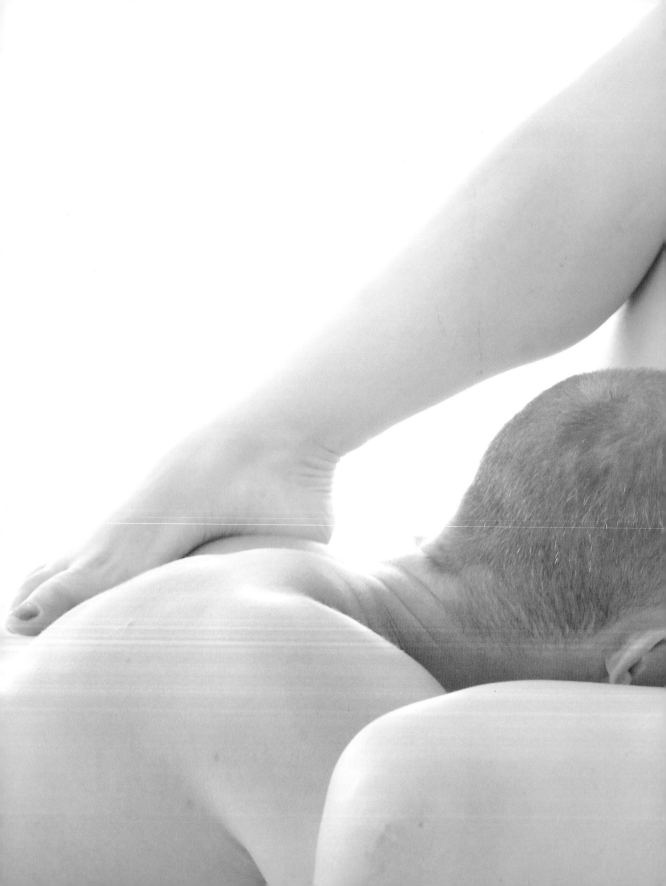

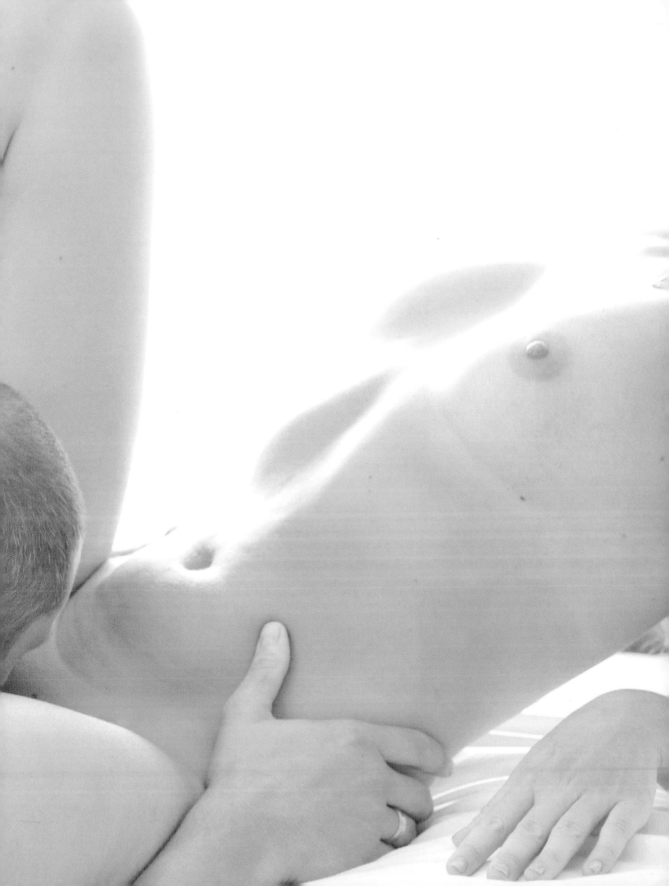

Dine and Dash

This scenario is particularly good if your gal is at all self-conscious about feeling her freshest as you settle in for a sweet treat. It will also add a nice kick to your evening. The next time you're going out for dinner, tell her you'd like to enjoy a quick appetizer at home before you leave. Ask her to meet you in the bedroom after her shower wearing just her robe or a towel. This will put her in a sexy frame of mind as she lathers up. Once she's freshly showered and you're both in the bedroom, set your alarm clock or your cellphone alarm and spend a minute going down on her. Don't waste any time on extracurricular activity like kissing or caressing and don't worry about getting her off. Stop when the alarm goes off and tell her to get dressed or you'll miss your dinner reservation. Enjoy your evening out (though you may find she wants to go home early).

AT YOUR FINGERTIPS

Fluffy towel or bathrobe for her

Alarm clock

Read My Lips

As she's curled up comfortably reading a book, kneel on the floor in front of her, gently pull her legs out from under her and lift her skirt or remove her pants, leaving her panties on. Tell her to read her book aloud to you while you kiss your way up and down her thighs for a minute or so. Lightly press your open mouth against her and exhale your hot breath through her panties. Kiss her softly through her underwear. Go back to kissing her thighs. Don't let her stop reading the entire time. Pull her panties aside and trace a few figure eights around her clitoris with your tongue. Stop, lift your head up, kiss her fully on the mouth, give her a wink that says "We'll have to finish this some other time," and tell her to go back to what she was doing.

> 66 Describe how beautiful and sexy she looks as she gets more and more turned on. 99

One Hour or Less

Die-ing for It

Keep dice in your bedside table so you can indulge in this adults-only game before lights out or before getting out of bed on a Sunday morning. Pull out one die and have her roll it. Set the timer to whatever number she rolls (use your cell phone if you don't have a timer handy), and lavish her with that many minutes of oral sex. When the time is up, have her roll the die again. Set the timer and spend that many minutes kissing her mouth and breasts. Go back and forth between oral sex and making out for as many rounds as it takes to get her off. Or try this variation: To make TV more interesting, have a single die next to you as you watch your favourite show. Pick a secret word (unless you want tongue-lash, you might want to avoid common words like "the" or "and") and, every time the word comes up, pause your show (if you don't already have a PVR, here's a great excuse to get one!), have her roll the die and bestow upon her the corresponding number of minutes of oral delight.

AT YOUR FINGERTIPS

Dice

Timer

Sweeten the Pot

Make Sunday morning breakfast in bed even sweeter. Hand her the paper and let her stay in bed while you get up and make breakfast—fresh-squeezed orange juice and pancakes with syrup. While you're juicing the oranges, take half an orange into the bedroom and ask her to tilt her head back, open her mouth and close her eyes. Squeeze some fresh orange juice directly into her mouth. After she swallows the deliciously sweet juice, follow up with a deep, long, soft kiss. Go back to the kitchen and finish making breakfast (if your culinary skills aren't up to snuff, pop a couple of frozen waffles in the toaster). Set up a tray with the orange juice, pancakes and a pitcher of maple syrup (go for the real stuff) and take it to her.

AT YOUR FINGERTIPS

Fresh oranges and juicer

Pancakes

Fresh maple syrup

As you enjoy your breakfast together, dip your finger into the maple syrup and run it over her lips (yes, the ones on her face). When she's done eating, put the tray aside, pull down the covers and remove her bottoms. Place a towel or cloth napkin underneath her bum to protect your sheets. Reach over and dip your finger into the syrup and let it drizzle over her clitoris. Lap it up by placing your tongue flat against the base of her clitoris and licking upward as if you were slowly licking an ice cream cone from bottom to top. Repeat.

- - - - - - - - - - - - - - - - - - - -

Quick Tip:
Hold the Sugar

If she's prone to yeast infections and therefore nervous about having something sugary dripped down there, trickle a glass of water over her clitoris instead.

- - - - - - - - - - - - - - - - - - - -

Sensational Taste!

Keep things exciting by alternating extreme sensations while you go down on her. Start by spending some time kissing to get her fired up. Before you head downtown, tell her you'll be back in a minute. Let her curiosity and excitement build as you head off to the kitchen to fetch a glass of ice cubes and a cup of hot water. Tell her to close her eyes, and place the glass of ice cubes and the cup of hot water beside the bed, out of her sight but within reaching distance for you (on the floor beside the bed should work just fine). Work your way down to her sweet spot, planting soft kisses along her tummy and hipbones as you do. Plant a few long, flat, slow, ice-cream licks from the bottom of her vulva all the way up and over her clitoris. Point your tongue and use the tip to circle her clitoris a few times. Go back to long, flat licks bottom to top followed by several short licks from the bottom of her clitoris to the top (like you're licking a mini ice cream cone, over and over, from bottom to top).

AT YOUR FINGERTIPS

Ice cubes

Cup of hot water

Towel

As she's getting into it, discreetly reach over, grab an ice cube and pop it into your mouth. Place the ice cube firmly between your teeth so it protrudes slightly from your lips. Holding it like this, slide the ice cube up and down between her labia. As the heat from her vagina and your mouth melts the ice, use your tongue to push the ice cube inside of her. The sudden coldness may cause her to gasp a little. Use this distraction to lean over and take a mouthful of water (it should have cooled enough by now, but if it's still too hot for your mouth, it's too hot for her preciousness and you need to let it cool some more). With the ice still melting inside her, press your mouth against her and release the water, letting the warm liquid gush over her entire vulva. Once she's accustomed to that sensation, slip her vagina another ice cube. Follow this with more warm water. The alternating sensations of hot and cold will keep her vagina guessing and interested. If you tire of the ice cube/water trick (or you think her vagina would like to try something new), try experimenting with other sensations. There are flavoured lubricants that warm up when you blow on them; drip some over her clitoris, breathe heavily and watch things heat up. Try popping a strong mint, like an Altoid, in your mouth while you are performing oral sex to create an intense tingling sensation. Or if you really want to rock her world, remember Pop Rocks? You can still buy them.

All Night

All You Can Eat

Oral pleasure is often enjoyed as a quick snack before dinner. Well, tonight I want you to give her the full meal deal. Make cunnilingus the appetizer, the main course *and* the dessert. Tell her you'll be her server, she is not to tip you and you're sorry, but intercourse isn't even on the menu.

Quick Tip:
Rub Her the Right Way
A little scruff can add some friction for sure, but twenty minutes of scruff is probably more friction than she's looking for. Be sure to shave before, uh, dinner.

You'll probably be most comfortable dining in the bedroom, but wherever you choose to chow down, create some atmosphere with candles and music. Make sure she's comfy and warm. Maybe start her off with a glass of wine, followed by lots of kissing and compliments. Nibble your way down her neck. Dust her shoulders with kisses. When a woman has her breasts kissed or nibbled in just the right way, it sends electric currents all the way down to her sex. Take your time here. Treat her breasts like you've just seen them for the first time and let your mouth explore them like Columbus discovering America. Plant light, feathery kisses along the soft underside of each breast and around the sides. Purse your wet lips around one nipple and pause for a few seconds until she feels the current running between her hardening nipple and your mouth. Slowly pull your lips away, and, as you do, swirl the firm tip of your tongue around the nipple. Alternate sensations from soft and gentle to sharp and intense. After a few soft licks of her nipple, clasp it very gently between your teeth to graze it as you pull away.

Quick Tip:
Go with the Flow
Cunnilingus need not be off limits during her period. Have her wash up beforehand and, if she's comfortable using tampons, insert a fresh one. If she's not a fan of tampons, she can use something called the Keeper, a rubber cup that is inserted deep inside the vagina against her cervix to catch her menstrual flow. Another option is a dental dam, a rectangular piece of latex available at most sex shops (or you can make your own from a regular condom by cutting off the tip and slicing it along one side so you can flatten it out) that you can hold in place while you go down on her.

Kiss your way down her body. Keep the electricity firing with light kisses down her arms and across her tummy. Lightly flick your tongue back and forth along her hipbones. If she's still wearing underwear, slide your tongue under the waistband and leg openings. Press your mouth against her undies and send your hot breath through the fabric. Pull them to one side and, using a flat, strong tongue, give her one long lick from bottom to top. Cover her up again. Go back to kissing her hips and tummy. Plant light kisses along the entire length of her inner thighs.

Slowly remove her panties (use your teeth to add some playful, animal flair) and take in the intoxicating smell of her vulva. Tell her how much it turns you on. She may be self-conscious about how she smells and tastes, so this reassurance that you're turned on by her scent will help her to relax and enjoy herself—it may even turn her on.

As you get into it, keep things wet. Your saliva and her wetness should provide plenty of natural lubricant, but don't hesitate to try adding a flavoured lubricant, especially on her clitoris. Lube will create a slick barrier between your tongue and her clit, adding extra slippery friction that will feel great for her. Or have a glass of water handy and take a sip every so often, letting some of the cool liquid trickle out as you work your magic with your tongue. As a general rule, long slow licks tend to be more welcome early on, while intense, firmer, faster licks usually work better the more turned on she is. But she'll appreciate

a variety of tongue action, from long, flat, soft licks to firmer licks, sideways licks and up-and-down licks. The key is to vary your tongue movements, but not to the point of being scattered. It's good to settle in once in a while. Think of a cat licking itself, working an area over and over again before moving on.

Quick Tip:
Detail-Oriented

When your partner asks if you like something they're doing, rather than responding with a simple "Yeah, that feels good," use the opportunity to give more specific feedback, framed positively, of course: "I love what you're doing with your fingers, especially when you do X," whatever "X" represents in your personal preference file.

The clitoris is her most sensitive bit (that's why it comes with that handy little hood) and unless she is very aroused and close to orgasm, too much direct stimulation of the little guy with your tongue can be, well, too much, too soon. As she becomes more aroused, her clitoris will swell and come out of its little shell (again, every woman is different and some women's become more evident than others). When it does, press your tongue, flat and slightly firm, at the base of the clitoris and lick upward along the underside of the

Quick Tip: Change Positions

Consider approaching oral sex from different angles. This will change how oral sex feels for her and give you both a fresh perspective. Certain positions give her more control. Others put you in the driver's seat. Some are more comfortable than others—I'd recommend these because the more comfortable she is, the more she'll be able to relax and enjoy herself, and the more comfy you are, the longer you'll be able to hang out without having to worry you'll end up in a neck brace. You don't have to stick to one position. If you do switch, watch your timing so as not to interrupt a crucial moment. You also don't want her to worry that you're moving because you're bored or to make her think she's taking too long. Stay enthusiastic. Before you switch positions, give her a look that says "If you liked that, wait until you see what I have in store for you next." Better yet, actually say this to her in your best playful, sexy voice. Consult "Playbook F: Changing Your Perspective" on pages 130–33 for suggestions.

clitoral shaft with long, steady licks from bottom to top. Point your tongue and run it in circles around her clitoris. Gently purse your lips over her clitoris and slide it in and out of your mouth (like you're giving her a miniature blow job!). Pull her clitoral hood back by stretching the skin taut around it. Curl your tongue into a tube (not everyone can do this), and slide it up and down her entire erect clitoris.

Most of the nerve endings inside her vagina are concentrated in the first couple of inches, conveniently about the length of your tongue. With your tongue firm and pointed, slide it into her vagina and swirl it in circles just inside the entrance. Now mix things up. Run your flat tongue from the bottom all the way up along the underside of her clitoris. Start from the bottom again and, every few trips up, stop along the way, point your tongue and slide the tip in and

out of her vagina a few times before you continue your journey up the entire length. Repeat.

After you've set up camp for a while and enjoyed gobbling up your favourite treat, supplement your tongue with some delicious extras. Fingers and toys can fill in when your tongue gets tired or if a leg cramp forces you to shift positions. They will also allow you to serve her a whole new array of tasty sensations. Even something as simple as running your fingers through her pubic hair or lightly tugging it while you're going down on her can send lovely shivers through her nether region. As she becomes more aroused, slip one or two fingers inside her vagina, sliding them in and out as you're licking her clitoris. Because fingers are slimmer than most penises and most of the nerves in her vagina are in the first couple of inches, this will be most effective if your hand is facing palm up and your fingers are curved to make contact with the front inside wall of her vagina as you slide in and out. This will also stimulate the G-spot area I referred to in the "Hand Job for Her" section and may cause her to, well—how to put this politely?—experience a physical release. You might find this incredibly sexy and satisfying (just make sure you don't articulate this agenda or she'll feel pressure to deliver), but not every guy enjoys a female-ejaculation face wash.

- -

Quick Tip:
In Focus

Pay close attention to her body language to help clue you in to when she's getting close to orgasm. If she's quiet and still, this doesn't necessarily mean she's not enjoying what you're doing. She may just be trying to concentrate on the sensations so she can get where she wants to be. If she's giving you the "don't stop what you're doing or I'll kill you" head grab (she can get away with this because there's less risk of choking than when you do it while she's going down on you) combined with the tensing of her entire body, don't stop what you're doing. Don't look up. Don't slow down. Just focus and keep a steady rhythm going.

- -

Instead of fingers, try using a sex toy—a dildo or phallic-shaped vibrator will work best—to penetrate her while your tongue is busy savouring her clitoris. They even make dildos that you can strap to your chin, if you can get over the visual without laughing, so you can penetrate her hands-free while going down on her. Warning: My experience with these is that, unless you have a very talented chin, you'll have little control over the dildo. They also make small vibrators that can be attached to your tongue to provide extra vibration while you go down on her. Again, in my experience, this works better in theory than in practice because as flexible as your tongue is, it doesn't have the dexterity that your hands do. If you want to add vibration during oral stimulation, it's more effective to hold a small vibrating egg against her clitoris while you're lapping at her lovely lady parts. Hold the vibrator steady against her clitoris, moving it in slow circles every few seconds to avoid numbness. Pulse the vibrator on and off (or use one with preset pulsing patterns). Then keep it steady again. While you're doing this, keep plying her labia with long licks of your flat tongue.

Getting her to orgasm with your mouth takes some dedication. The more you practise, the better you'll get. Eventually, you'll learn to read her body signals and get a sense of when she's getting close. Generally, the closer a woman is to orgasm, the more consistent she needs your tongue to be. This is not the time to suddenly switch gears. If her hips are several inches above the bed, her toes are curled and she's got you in a thigh headlock, you need to keep doing what you're doing. Yes, I know your tongue feels like it's about to fall off and breathing is a challenge, but hang in there, partner. You're almost home!

Unless you want to torture her a little. Which can also be fun. When she is on the brink, pull away, count to five and go back to what you were doing. Bring her back to the brink, stop again, count to five and go back. See how long you can keep her on the edge before finally pushing her over.

> 66 She'll appreciate a variety of tongue action, from long, flat, soft licks to firmer licks, sideways licks and up-and-down licks. The key is to vary your tongue movements. 99

Once she comes (she may not, and that's okay as long as she enjoyed the ride), hold your tongue flat against her clitoris and the opening of her vagina. Give her a few long, slow, firm licks. Let her feel the connection to your soft, wet mouth as she rides the waves of orgasm. Your wet mouth on her as she climaxes will feel heavenly. Keep licking. If your fingers aren't inside her

already, intensify the sensations by sliding one (or two) inside as she's coming and thrusting through her orgasm. If you're still using a vibrator, reduce the speed and circle it lazily around her clitoris once or twice before turning it off completely. When she comes back down to earth, leave her with a few slow, flat-tongued licks and a soft kiss on the lips (yes, her vagina's lips) as your way of saying thank you.

Quick Tip:
Staying Power

Tongues can't provide the same pressure or move as fast as fingers or toys, so getting her to orgasm may take a little longer. Most women take an average of at least fifteen to twenty minutes to orgasm from oral sex. If you don't think your mouth can last that long, add stimulation from your fingers or a vibrator against her clitoris to help get her to orgasm.

PLAYBOOK F
CHANGING HIS PERSPECTIVE

BACK TO BASICS

Description: A tried and true classic. She lies on her back with her knees bent and her feet flat on the bed. You lie on your stomach with your face between her legs. You can curl your arms under her bum cheeks and hook your hands around either hip for stability and support. Place a pillow under her bum to raise her pelvis so it is in line with your mouth.

Pros: Comfy for her. Also, if she masturbates like this, it will be a familiar position for her to achieve orgasm, potentially making it easier to get her there. A pillow under her hips will give your mouth better access. In this position, you can also lift your head and get a great view of her tummy, breasts and face and give her a big, wet smile to show her what a good time you're having.

Cons: After a while, your neck will start to feel like you've been sitting too close to the stage all night. The pillow under her bottom will help but, if your neck starts to kink, let your hands step in for a moment and maybe do a few neck curls before putting your mouth back to work.

Variation: To make her vulva even more accessible, she pulls her knees up toward her chest, letting her legs fall open and tucking her hands under her knees to help hold them up. You may find it more comfortable to kneel and lower your mouth to her vagina using your arms as support. This way, your neck will be more aligned with your spine, alleviating potential neck strain.

SIT, GIRL, SIT

Description: She sits with her bum shifted forward to the edge of the bed—or chair, countertop, table—with her legs spread, feet resting flat on the floor if they can reach. You kneel on the floor between her legs so that your face is at pelvis level. Place a pillow under your knees for comfort. Depending on the height of whatever she's sitting on, you may need to lower your bum onto your heels. You can also sit cross-legged or with your legs stretched out in front of you and a pillow under your butt.

Pros: You don't have to tilt your head, so it's easier on your neck. She can look down and get a bird's-eye view of the action and you can look up and make eye contact. You can reach up and touch her breasts (as well as her inner thighs or any other body parts within reach) while going down on her.

Cons: She may find it difficult to stay perched on the edge of whatever she's sitting on for a long time. A pillow under her butt can help alleviate this. While you can easily access her clitoris in this position, her actual vagina is facing down, so you'll have a harder time reaching it with your tongue.

Variations:
- If she's sitting on the bed, she can lie back with her butt hanging slightly over the edge, making it easier to access her entire vulva with your mouth.
- Depending on how flexible she is, have her sit on an armchair and draw her knees up, placing one foot on either arm, further opening herself up to you. If she can't get her feet on the arms, she can pull her legs up and plant her feet wide apart on either side of the chair's seat. Or she can hook her legs over your shoulders, allowing her to gain some control by pulling you closer when she wants more pressure.

THE FACE PLANT
Description: You lie on your back on the bed or floor. She kneels, straddling your head so that she is perfectly positioned to lower herself over your mouth. For support, she can lean back and place her hands on the bed or lean forward and place her hands on the wall or bed frame.

Pros: She can move her pelvis back and forth and up and down across your tongue, giving her more control, grinding into you if she wants more pressure and pulling away if she wants a lighter touch. You get a wonderful lesson in what she likes without having to do or say anything. You also get a great view of her upper body writhing around on top of you.

Cons: It's hard to move your tongue with a vagina sitting on it. She can lift her pelvis slightly so that you get a chance to show her some of your own moves. Place a pillow under

The Face Plant

In this position, she can move around and make sure you're hitting the right spots.

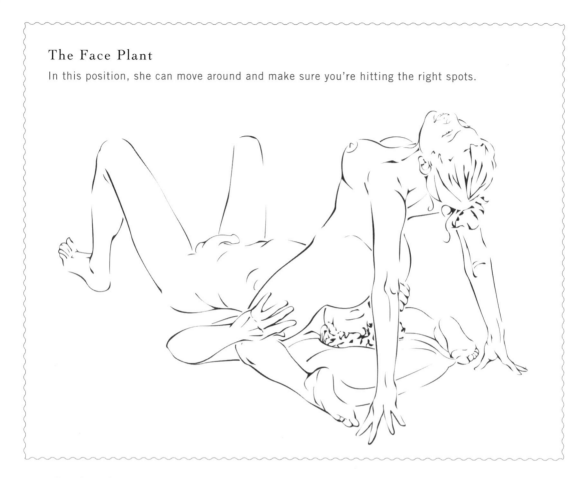

your head so that you don't have to strain your neck to reach. Breathing might be an issue if she gets really turned on and starts grinding more intensely against your mouth. Luckily, in this position your hands are free to wave a white flag or grab her hips and gently lift to let her know you need to come up for air.

Variations:

- She kneels facing your feet and leans forward with her hands flat on the bed to support her upper body. You get a great rear view of her wiggling bottom as she slides her vagina over your mouth and tongue. Elevate your head with a pillow so you can comfortably taste her from behind.

- You lie on your back across the bed with your head dangling slightly over the edge. She stands facing the bed and positions herself over your mouth (if your bed isn't the right height, find something that is). You can move your mouth more easily because your head isn't pinned to the bed and she can still move her pelvis back and forth across your mouth while getting a great view of your hot bod.

REAR VIEW

Description: She kneels on all fours or leans forward on her upper arms with her butt in the air. Depending on her height and yours, you can kneel, sit cross-legged or sit with your legs stretched out in front of you between her legs so your mouth is level with her vagina.

Pros: She enjoys the varied sensations of feeling your tongue and mouth from a completely different angle. You get a great rear view while going down on her. If she enjoys vaginal penetration with your tongue, this puts you in the best position to fulfill that desire.

Cons: With you back there and her facing forward, there's little opportunity to make eye contact. While this position gives you great access to her vagina, unless you have a Gene Simmons tongue, you're probably not going to have much luck reaching her clitoris from this angle. This problem is easily solved by using your fingers or a vibrator against her clit as your tongue has its way with her vagina.

Variations:
- If she gets tired on all fours, she can lie on her stomach with her legs spread and a pillow or two under her pelvis to raise her bum so you can still access her vagina from behind. You lie on your stomach between her legs and bury your mouth between them. If you need something to hold on to for stability, you can curl your arms under and around her thighs and use your hands to spread her butt cheeks for better access to her vagina.
- She kneels on all fours (or supporting herself on her upper arms with her butt raised in the air) at the edge of the bed while you sit comfortably behind her in a chair.
- You sit in a chair as she stands with her back to you and her legs spread on either side of you. She bends over at the waist, hands on the floor if she can reach or braced against the wall or on the seat of another chair in front of her, giving you front-row access.

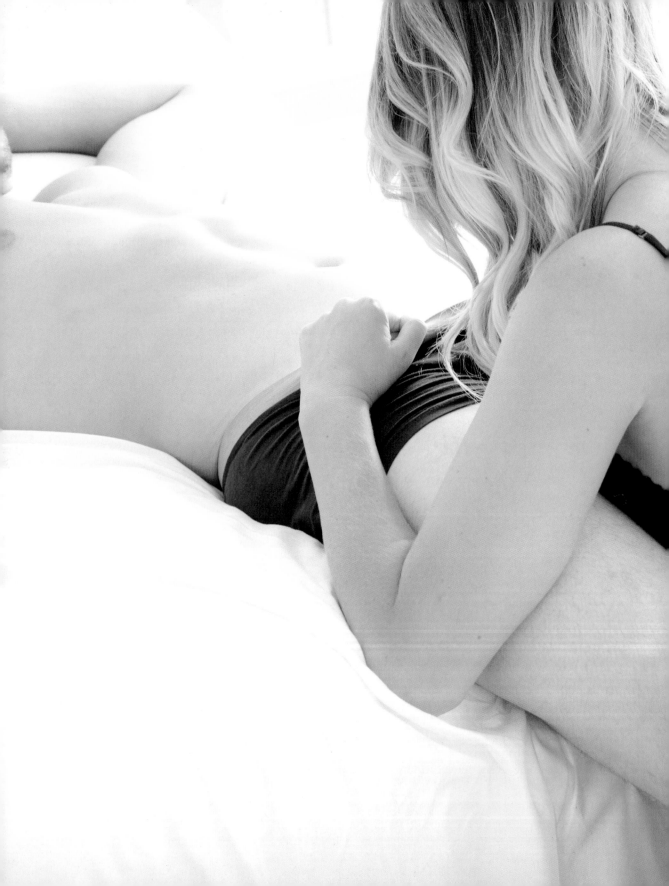

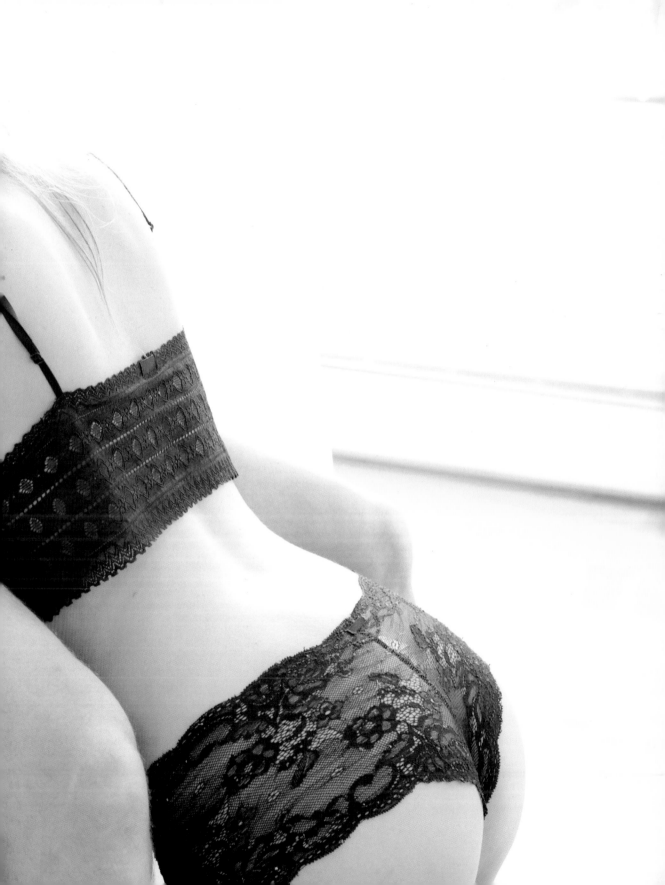

FELLATIO

Being able to give him a mind-blowing blow job is the time-strapped girl's little black dress. You don't have to put a lot of time or thought into it (unless you want to—more on that in a minute) and it always makes you look great. And most guys love them! Blow jobs are convenient. He doesn't even have to take off his pants. You could put this book down right now, lead him into the bedroom, bathroom or any other space where you know you won't be disturbed for a few minutes, and give him a blow job.

Pop culture would have you believe that your guy isn't fussy about his fellatio—he's just happy to get some. But guys like a gal who knows what she's doing down there. And if you take the time to learn what he likes and try new things, it will make him feel like you really care about him and his pleasure.

> 66 Being able to give him a mind-blowing blow job is the time-strapped girl's little black dress. 99

Fellatio can be fast and dirty or slow and seductive. Dropping to your knees while he's cooking dinner is a nice way to surprise him (just make sure he's not cooking anything that splatters). A long, leisurely blow job while he's comfortably reclined on a soft bed with some great music and lighting is a great way to show him all your best moves and drive him to the edge and back . . . several times . . . until he's begging for release. You will make him feel like the luckiest man alive.

TIME to PLAY

Five Minutes or Less

Visual Display

Look him in the eye, take his finger in your mouth and give him a "finger job." Also works with popsicles or any other suggestively shaped food item.

A Special Goodbye Kiss

After he's dressed and before he leaves for work, tell him to drop his pants, take his soft penis in your mouth and make it hard using your mouth. Pull his pants back up, kiss him and tell him to have a great day. When he gives you that pleading look and begs you to finish the job, tell him he'll just have to wait because you have to run. Oh, don't worry, he'll survive.

Making Quick Work of It

Most guys can get off pretty quickly from oral sex. If you don't have a lot of time, preliminaries can be kept to a minimum. Just make sure your intention is more

"Mmm, I can't wait to get my lips on that fine thing" than "Okay, fine, let's get this over with." Then drop to your knees, tell him you're going to see if you can get him off in under a minute, unzip him and take him in your mouth. If you don't make it, let him finish the job himself while you watch. Then tell him you'll just have to try harder next time.

One Hour or Less

Stick Shift

Blow jobs, like hand jobs, are fairly portable. Use this advantage and take your blow job on the road. A bathroom stall, an alleyway or a remote corner in the park are just a few exciting places you could get away with it. Or how about literally taking your blow job on the road? When's the last time you went down on him in the front seat of the car? Next time you're en route somewhere, keep your eye out for a dead-end road or a deserted rest stop. When you spot a likely place, ask him to pull over. If he asks why, tell him you feel like a snack. When he notices there isn't anywhere to eat nearby, raise your eyebrows and give him a sneaky smile to let him know what you mean.

Blow Job with a Cherry on Top

Tell him to get naked and wait for you on the bed. You might want to lay a towel or a plastic sheet under him because things will get messy. Head off to the kitchen and fill a tray with all the fixin's for a chocolate sundae—ice cream, chocolate sauce, whipped cream and, of course, a cherry. Oh, and why not toss on an apron and some heels to give the whole thing a nice, naughty 1950s pin-up girl vibe? Bring the tray into the bedroom and make a big production out of turning your baby's bippy into a delectable ice cream sundae that you then slowly and seductively devour one sweet and creamy mouthful at a time.

AT YOUR FINGERTIPS

Old towel or plastic sheet

Chocolate sundae ingredients

Apron

High heels

Hands Off

Forbid him from touching himself (or you) while you spend at least fifteen minutes using your tongue everywhere on his body, except where he'll be begging you—from the very core of that same body—to use it. Kiss his shoulders, his neck, his mouth. Run your tongue along the inside of his thighs, along his hips and across his nipples. If he tries to touch himself or you, tell him you'll stop altogether if he doesn't behave. When he looks like his head is about to spin around on his neck, use your mouth to play his organ until he sings with pleasure.

All Night

Day-Blow

Indulge your baby with a day-long blow job. Start in the morning by texting him that he's in for a delicious treat tonight. In the middle of the day, ask him how he feels about you devoting the entire evening to his pleasure. When he gets home, kiss him deeply when he walks in the door, sliding your hand down the front of his pants. Sit him down to his favourite dinner and make a point of suggestively licking your fingers and your lips while you eat. After dinner, tell him to take a shower, get dressed and meet you in the bedroom. While he's showering, slip into something sexy and wait for him on the bed.

When he comes in, ask him to join you on the bed. Spend some time kissing. Shower him with lots of compliments. Tell him you loved how he made you laugh earlier in the day. Growling in his ear, tell him you've been thinking about this all day and that you plan to drive him absolutely bonkers. While he still has his pants on, slide your hand along the inside of his thigh, across his groin and back down the inside of his other thigh. As you remove his shirt, kiss your way down his neck and shoulders. Nibble on his ear. Whisper how you're dying to feel his gorgeous hunk of manhood in your warm, wet mouth. Unless your guy really doesn't like to have his nipples touched or kissed, don't neglect them

on the way down. Run your tongue around the outside of each nipple. Grab a nipple gently between your teeth and close your soft mouth over it. Pull away slowly so your teeth graze his nipple. Trickle light kisses down his "happy trail," the strip of skin or hair below his belly button. Look into his eyes as you slowly undo his pants and slide them off, one leg at a time.

> ❝Growling in his ear, tell him you've been thinking about this all day and that you plan to drive him absolutely bonkers.❞

Don't remove his briefs (or boxers or whatever he wears) yet. Make him wait for it. The tease will make it that much more delicious when he finally gets to feel your lovely mouth on his penis. Place your mouth against his underwear and blow warm air against him through the fabric. Run your tongue all along the inside of his waistband as you look up at him to convey "I've got you where I want you and I'm enjoying this." Go back to kissing his neck and shoulders. Turn around and grind your bottom into his lap. Keep up the tease as long as you can.

After you slowly peel off his underwear, keep up the crazy making. If he's already erect, tease him by rubbing your breasts along the shaft of his penis, followed by a long lick with a flat soft tongue from the base of his testicles along the underside of his shaft and all the way to the tip of his penis. Go back to kissing his happy trail or along his inner thighs (heck, why not start at his ankles?) and make your way back up to his penis. If he's not erect when you get his underwear off (hey, it happens), take his soft penis entirely into your mouth. Swirl your tongue around the tip and slide his entire penis in and out as you feel it grow bigger in your mouth, until you've got his full attention.

- -

Quick Tip:
Comfort Zone

As with him going down on you, perform-ing oral sex in different positions changes your access and your view as well as how it feels for him. And again, if you're physically uncomfortable, you'll be more anxious to get it over with—no fun—so find a position that feels good. Consult "Playbook G: Changing Your Viewpoint" on pages 144–47 for ideas.

- -

Having his penis in your juicy, warm mouth feels a bit like having it in your vagina—that is, if your vagina had a tongue. To get a sense of how your tongue feels on his penis, practise on your own finger. Swirl a soft, semi-flat tongue around the tip, then flick a pointy, firm tongue on the inside of your finger to get a sense of what it feels like when you flick the under-side of the head of his penis. Engulf your entire finger in your mouth and slide it up and down, varying the pressure.

With the real thing in front of you, keep in mind that the most sensitive spot on your guy's penis is the head or glans, in particular the frenulum, the underside of the tip where the head meets the shaft. Apply light flicks with the tip of your tongue to this area. Twirl the length of your tongue around the entire head. Use long, slow licks with a flat tongue up the entire length of the under-side of his penis all the way to the tip. Do the same using short, quick flicks of your tongue. If he's uncircumcised, pull the fore-skin up over the head, slip it the tongue and swirl your way around the head. Make sure your lips are nice and wet (use flavoured lube if you want more wetness). Rub the head of his penis around your lips as if you were applying lipstick. Try taking him in your mouth as far as you can, just once or twice, and then move back to the outlying regions, kissing his thighs or his hipbones.

Place your mouth over the head of his penis and suck it in and out. Every few strokes, slide your mouth down as far as it will go. Alternate shallow mouth strokes with deep mouth strokes. If you are afraid to trigger your gag reflex, you can create the feeling of taking him deep into your mouth by using your hands along with your mouth. Circle your fist around the base of his penis, using saliva or lube to make it wet and slippery. Slide your mouth over the head of his penis and down the shaft as far as it is comfortable, sliding your hand up to meet it if necessary. Move your fist and your mouth in tandem. Slide your mouth up and off his penis followed by your hand sliding up the shaft. Reverse and slide your hand down the shaft followed by your mouth. Repeat. This mouth/hand combo mimics the warm, wet feeling of being deep in your mouth but allows you to stop him from thrusting too deep.

- -

Quick Tip:
Put a Ring on It

A cock ring is a ring made out of leather, vinyl or rubber that you can get at any sex shop. Place it around the base of his penis before he becomes hard to intensify his erection while you go down on him.

- -

Once you've given his penis a good licking, move down and show his boys some love. Flutter your eyelashes against his testicles. Shower them with some feathery kisses. Gently draw one and then the other into your mouth. Run your tongue around his entire package and then slide it all the way back up the shaft.

From here, his penis is your oyster. Get creative. Here are some ideas:

• Hum a little tune as you slide your mouth sideways up and down the entire length.

• Purse your lips and blow cool air up and down the length of his penis. Alternate this with hot breath up and down his shaft.

• Place the shaft of his penis against your neck and purr so he can feel the vibration.

• Slide your mouth about halfway down his penis and create a seal over the head. Lengthen your tongue and swirl the entire thing around the head of his penis, keeping your lips tight around it. Suck up and down for a few strokes, then go back to swirling with your tongue.

• Curl your tongue and slip the tip of his penis inside, so that the underside is lying against the flat of your tongue. Use your upper lip to hold the tip of his "hot dog" firmly inside your tongue "hot dog bun." Slide your tongue in and out of your mouth, keeping a firm connection between his hot dog and your bun as you do.

• A light scrape of the teeth over the tip of his penis or down the shaft and along the testicles can feel really great. If he looks nervous, stick to using your tongue and lips. If you want to avoid teeth-to-penis contact altogether, cover your teeth with your lips as you slide your mouth down the shaft.

• Put an ice cube in your mouth when you go down on him or while you suck on his testicles. Remove the ice cube and blow hot breath on his penis and testicles.

• Hold a vibrator next to your tongue as you suck on his penis. Focus the vibration on the sensitive underside of the tip, run the vibrator along the shaft and circle his boys with it.

• Put on some tingly or minty lip balm and then go down on him.

• Use your mouth with some of the tips from "Playbook E: Tricky Moves" on pages 113–15.

Don't make your man feel as if your main purpose is to get him to orgasm. Since you've got the time, you might as well both enjoy the ride. When, however, you decide you want to take him over the finish line, you'll want to settle into a good steady pumping rhythm. With your hand circled around the base of his penis, slide your mouth over the head of his penis and move your mouth up and down. Keep your lips nice and tight

around his penis to create gentle suction. If you like, slide your hand up along the shaft right behind your mouth and slide it back down again as you slide your mouth down. This will keep the suction going and make it feel like one long, warm, moist sucking tube. I know, hot. Anyway, once you get a good rhythm going and feel his thighs tense and his breath quicken, you'll sense he's getting close. If you generally have trouble knowing when he's about to come, establish a signal beforehand that he can use to let you know. A simple tap on the shoulder, for example.

- -

Quick Tip:
Go Deep

Deep-throating is one of those things we can blame on porn. Whether you choose to go there is entirely up to you. If you want to go there, here's a nifty trick. Lie on your back on the bed with your head hanging slightly over the edge. Have him stand at the edge of the bed facing you with his pelvis at your eye level (he may need to crouch or kneel, depending on his height and that of your bed). Direct his erect penis into your mouth. With your head upside down and tilted back in this way, your neck is elongated to create a straight line down your throat that allows for deep penetration without any gag reflex. It sounds weird, I know, but it works!

- -

Once he's at this point, it's crucial that you keep up a steady speed and rhythm in order to take him over the edge. If you find you have trouble bringing him to orgasm with your mouth, another option is to have him finish things off with his own hand while you lick and suck his testicles and compliment him on the view. As you get more familiar with his "tipping point"—that is, the moment before he is about to come—have some fun with it. As you feel him getting close, slow down whatever you're doing until he returns from the brink. Take him close to orgasm again, and then slow down again. Do this a few times and you'll significantly intensify his orgasm when you finally do let him come.

Yes, it can be hot for both of you, but I don't think any woman loves to swallow (despite what you see in porn). You might like the intimacy of it, or how happy it makes him, but let's be honest, it's not exactly like drinking a vanilla milkshake. If you can't bear to swallow, don't. Instead, compromise and have him come *near* your mouth. He gets the visual and you're spared the swallowing sensation. Another trick is to curl your tongue just as he's about to orgasm so that the head of his penis is hitting the underside of your tongue. That way, your tongue will block his ejaculate from shooting down your throat. Once he climaxes, slowly slide your mouth off his penis, giving the head a sweet goodbye kiss as you leave.

> 66 Flutter your eyelashes against his testicles. Shower them with some feathery kisses. 99

Quick Tip: Taste Test

Lots of guys have asked me if they can alter the taste of their semen through diet. Not surprisingly, no scientific studies have been done on how diet affects the taste of semen (or vaginal fluids for that matter, ladies), which is pretty understandable. Imagine the scene at the taste test: "Okay, there are three cups of semen in front of you, all from complete strangers who we've had on various diets. Ladies, please take a sip from each and describe the taste." Mmm, good. That being said, it's perfectly logical that the taste of both sperm and vaginal fluids would be affected by diet. You are what you eat, after all. And plenty of less-than-scientific suggestions are floating around out there. I've come across claims that alkaline-based foods such as meats and fish produce a buttery, fishy taste. Apparently, dairy products can really funk up your spunk. Citrus fruits, however, are rumoured to create a more bitter taste. And I've heard it suggested that you avoid cauliflower and broccoli, as well as foods heavy on garlic and onions, if you want to taste sweeter. Oh, and I love this one: Apparently beer sweetens your bodily fluids. But fellas, just be careful not to do so much flavour enhancing that you'll be too drunk to produce any delicious flavour-enhanced semen.

❦ Foreplay Cheat Sheet ❧

☐ Hug each other once a day for at least a minute. Hold hands when you're out together. Touch during regular conversation. Caress her cheek. Brush his arm.

☐ If you don't have time for a full-body massage, try a one-minute hand rub or a thirty-second shoulder rub.

☐ During masturbation or hand jobs, use lube or oil to increase sensation.

☐ Don't always masturbate the same way.

☐ When you're both tired and sex seems like too much effort, try masturbating together.

☐ Avoid intense, direct rubbing or licking of the clitoris until she is highly aroused or close to orgasm.

☐ Use a vibrator against her clitoris to bring her to orgasm quickly. Add penetration using your fingers, a dildo or a vibrator as you stimulate her clitoris.

☐ Use a firm grip when giving him a hand job. Keep your hand jobs from becoming predictable by experimenting with different strokes.

☐ Apply soft licks to his most sensitive spot, the underside of the tip of his penis where the head meets the shaft. Alternate shallow mouth strokes with deep mouth strokes.

☐ As you feel your partner getting close to orgasm, ramp up the intensity of your strokes while keeping the rhythm steady.

☐ Take your partner to the brink of orgasm, pause, then take them back to the brink. Repeat until you decide to grant them sweet release.

PLAYBOOK G
CHANGING YOUR VIEWPOINT

LAID BACK

Description: He lies on his back with his legs spread. You kneel between his legs with your bum resting on your heels and lower your mouth over his penis.

Pros: Comfy for him. You can make eye contact while you're going down on him. Your hands are free to guide his penis into your mouth and control the depth and speed.

Cons: Angle can be awkward and uncomfortable for her. Your legs may go to sleep after a while in this position.

Variations:

- You kneel to one side of him. This allows you to more easily lower your mouth onto his penis from above.
- He sits up with his back against the headboard or wall. You kneel beside him, resting your bum on your heels, and lower your head to his penis.
- He lies on his side. You lie on your side facing him and shift your body down so your mouth is in line with his penis and your hands are free to assist.

TAKE A STAND

Description: He stands. You kneel in front of him so that your mouth is level with his penis.

Pros: Handy if there's no bed to lie on. Your hands are free to control his thrusting and also to play with his testicles, run your fingers across his lower back, or massage his buttocks. Creates a submissive power dynamic that can be a turn-on.

Cons: The submissive power dynamic might be a turnoff. Can also be hard on your knees — kneeling on a pillow will help.

Variation: He stands in front of you while you sit in a chair facing him. This position eliminates the submissive element and allows you to approach his penis from the direction it is no doubt (or soon will be) pointing.

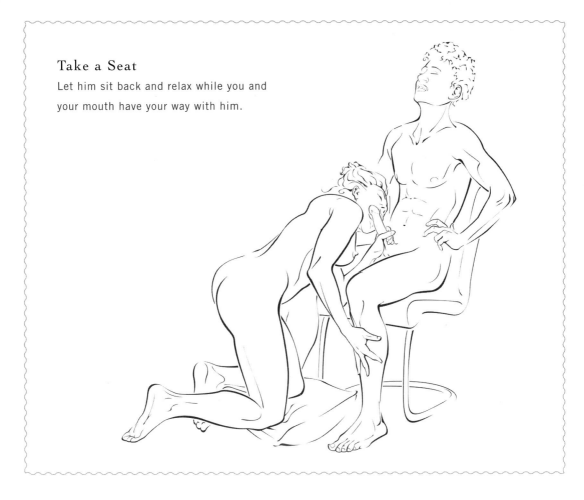

Take a Seat

Let him sit back and relax while you and
your mouth have your way with him.

TAKE A SEAT

Description: He sits on a chair (that way he can relax, watch TV . . . only kidding) or the edge of the bed with his knees spread. You kneel between his legs.

Pros: Comfy for him. Great for eye contact. You have great access to his penis and can also use your hands to caress his chest, arms and thighs.

Cons: Hard on your knees—a pillow will help with this.

Variation: He sits on a countertop so that you can stand up (depending on your height, you may need to bend your knees a little or plop a pillow or two under his butt to raise him up higher) while going down on him.

BRING HIM TO HIS KNEES

Description: He kneels upright on the bed with his legs spread. You kneel facing him with your bum resting on your heels or sit with your legs stretched out in between his and lower your mouth to his penis.

Pros: He gets a great view of you going down on him. He can play with your hair or occasionally lean down, gently pull your chin up toward him and kiss you on the mouth. You can raise your head and kiss his hips, stomach and torso.

Cons: If you're sitting, movement of your entire body is limited.

Variation: He kneels on all fours supporting his upper body on his hands or elbows while you lie comfortably on your back beneath him with your face in line with his pelvis. Place a pillow or two under your neck to raise your head and create a better angle for your mouth.

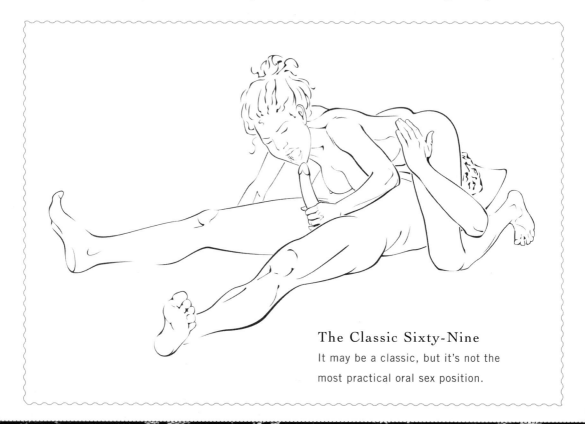

The Classic Sixty-Nine
It may be a classic, but it's not the most practical oral sex position.

A FEW WORDS ABOUT THE CLASSIC SIXTY-NINE

The sixty-nine is by far the most famous oral sex position, but it is also probably the least effective for giving each other great oral sex. To perform this, he lies on his back while you kneel on all fours on top of him in the opposite direction, so that your head is over his penis and your pelvis is over his mouth. You use one hand to support your upper body and the other to hold his penis while you go down on him as you lower your vagina to meet his mouth. Or the opposite. Okay, I'm already exhausted. And depending on your height difference, the necessary parts might not even line up, making things even more complicated.

Sure, the idea that you're pleasuring each other at the same time can be a turn-on, at least for a while. Most people find it hard to concentrate on both giving and receiving pleasure for a significant length of time, making this position rather inefficient, especially if time is an issue. If you like this position, you may both get more out of it if you take turns: You go down on him for a spell, he goes down on you. Kind of like riding a seesaw—a really hot seesaw.

A more comfortable variation on the sixty-nine is for both of you to lie on your sides in opposite directions so your head is in front of his penis and his head is lying on the inner thigh of your bottom leg. You can move your top knee down and rest on his shoulder for comfort. This doesn't give you the direct access to each other that the traditional sixty-nine does, but it can be a sweet and comfy way to enjoy mutual oral sex.

> **"You may both get more out of it if you take turns: You go down on him for a spell, he goes down on you."**

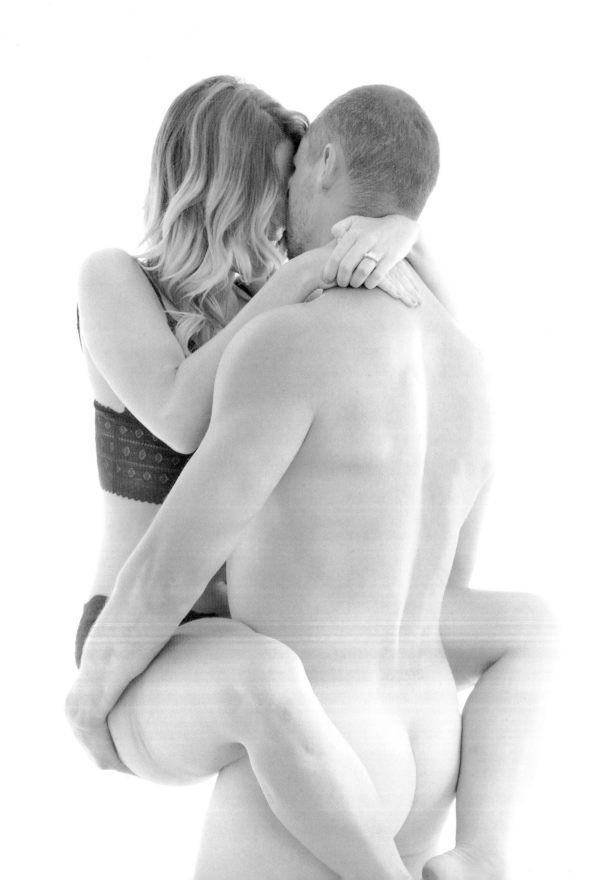

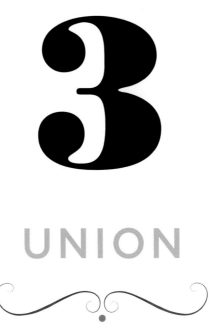

3

UNION

Bringing your bodies together in physical union is one of the most profound ways to connect as a couple. If you're in sync, you're like two pieces of a puzzle. That moment when you look into each other's eyes and he enters you can be intense, intimate and powerful. But if you don't keep intercourse fresh and exciting, that moment can lose its impact. If your intercourse becomes unsurprising and automatic, you will undoubtedly find yourself less inspired to make time for it. My goal is to show you how to give your lovemaking a much-needed kick in the butt, metaphorically, of course. I suggest, however, that you do other things to each other's butts. As a less orthodox form of union, anal sex can challenge you in new and stimulating ways both physically and emotionally. The amount of trust required and the new sensations you can experience through anal play can deepen your relationship and your connection. To complete the union trilogy, I encourage you to explore the spiritual side of sex through tantric practices that help you to be more present in your lovemaking, to open your heart and mind so you can connect on a more soulful level.

So, if you're ready to learn how to add a new thrust to your lovemaking or want to experiment with adding sex toys to your intercourse, keep reading. If you've never tried anal sex because you were intimidated, nervous or put off, this part will show you that you need not be any of those things and that there are many different ways to enjoy anal play. If anal sex is already part of your sexual repertoire, you're certain to find some new things to try. I end on a more mystical note and teach you how to take advantage of tantric sexual practices to intensify your emotional and spiritual connection during sex.

Time Challenge

If you have ten seconds . . .
While she's getting undressed, shower her bottom with kisses through her panties.

If you have two minutes . . .
Experiment with a few different sexual positions while fully clothed.

If you have five minutes . . .
Throw her on the bed for a quickie!

If you have fourteen minutes . . .
Massage each of his seven chakras.

If you have fifteen minutes . . .
Bring yourself close to orgasm with a vibrator while he strokes himself to orgasm. Have him enter you as you both climax.

If you have half an hour . . .
Sit naked facing each other and focus on syncing your breathing.

If you have an hour . . .
While you're having sex doggie-style, hold a vibrator against her backside.

If you have all night . . .
Take a candlelit bubble bath together. Afterward, get her to lie on the bed on her tummy and, using plenty of oil, massage her back and legs, working your way up to exploring her bottom with your fingers.

START WITH THE BASICS

Warm up the engine.

Unless it's a quickie, sex will be more intense and exciting if there's been lots of kissing and teasing first. And there is no such thing as quickie anal sex. No matter how turned on or eager you are, never ever rush into it. Bums generally like to be entered only when they are good and damn ready.

The wetter the better.

Supplement any intercourse (especially anal) with lube. It will feel good for both of you.

Let her clitoris in on the fun.

An estimated 70 percent of women don't come through penetration alone and need some kind of clitoral stimulation to climax.

Turn off your brain.

Don't let your head run the show. Whenever it interrupts with something critical or distracting, focus instead on the spiritual connection and the sexual energy flowing between your bodies.

Mix it up.

Don't do it in the same place or in the same way every time.

Let the love flow.

Open your hearts and focus on the emotional connection between the two of you.

Enjoy the journey.

Sure, orgasms are nice, but if you spend too much time worrying about coming, you won't be in the moment for all the other good stuff and, ironically, that will make it harder to come.

It's okay to laugh.

Like anything else, sex is less about getting it "right" than about being in the moment and enjoying yourselves. Besides, laughter is a wonderful way to connect.

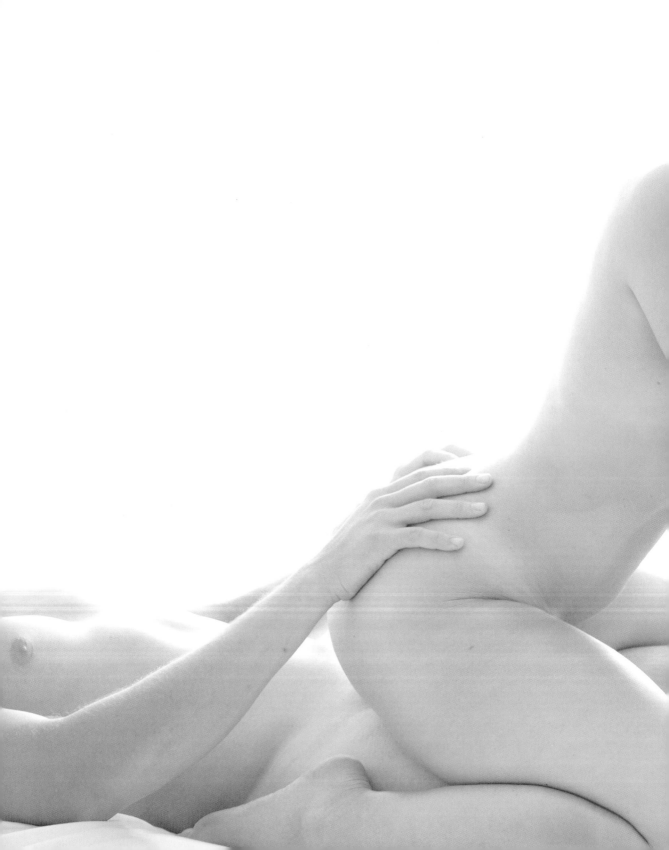

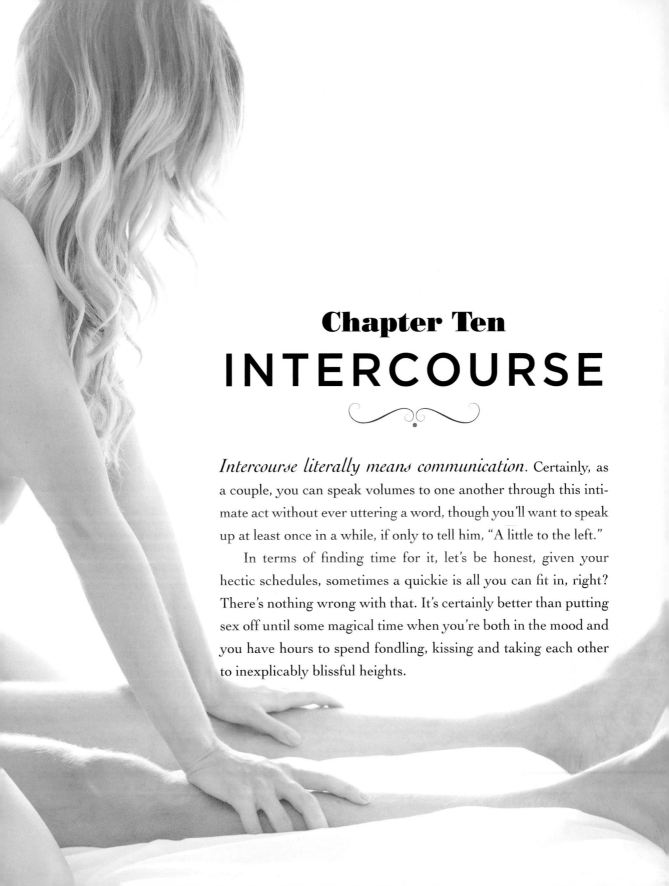

Chapter Ten
INTERCOURSE

Intercourse literally means communication. Certainly, as a couple, you can speak volumes to one another through this intimate act without ever uttering a word, though you'll want to speak up at least once in a while, if only to tell him, "A little to the left."

In terms of finding time for it, let's be honest, given your hectic schedules, sometimes a quickie is all you can fit in, right? There's nothing wrong with that. It's certainly better than putting sex off until some magical time when you're both in the mood and you have hours to spend fondling, kissing and taking each other to inexplicably blissful heights.

Besides, what could be more boring and predictable than having sex for the same length of time every time? Sometimes, the spontaneity of a quickie is just the kind of sexual shot in the arm you both need. That's right, contrary to common belief, guys aren't the only ones who like quickies. Women love them too. A good quickie has an element of excitement and surprise. It says that you feel so overcome with passion you just can't wait. What's not to love about that? Unfortunately, because of all the pressure to spend time on foreplay, a lot of guys feel guilty about quickies. Maybe that's part of the problem. If you're sneaking something guiltily, you'll probably seem guilty, and that will just annoy her. Occasionally she wants you to do away with all the trimmings, pin her against the hall table and get right down to business. No guilt.

When you do have time for a longer session that doesn't involve stopwatches and hall furniture, there's plenty you can do to keep intercourse electrifying and inspired that still doesn't require a lot of time or effort: A different thrust, a new position, an unfamiliar setting or maybe a sex toy are all uncomplicated ways to throw some new fuel onto the fire.

With a nice variety of intercourse options to choose from, you'll have something to suit every mood and time constraint. Just as learning new recipes makes you more excited about cooking, adding new items to your sex menu will get you more excited and drive you to make time for it, be it a lunchtime quickie or a drawn-out romantic affair complete with orgasms all around.

TIME to PLAY

Five Minutes or Less

Quick and Clean

Sex in the shower is a time-strapped couple's, um, wet dream. Showering together saves time and water (so you're doing your bit for the planet too!), and because you have to finish before the hot water runs out, you get right down to business. Cleanup is easy. Oh, and the sight of water splashing down your darlin's naked body as you get it on is pretty fricking hot too. Soap her breasts for a hot visual and some sexy caressing. Use your slippery wet hands to stroke him to erection. The trickiest part of shower sex is finding a workable position that won't land both of you on your soapy butts. If she's flexible and your heights match up, she can bend over at the waist and brace herself against the floor of the shower, the edge of the tub or the wall as you enter her from behind. Alternatively, if you can lift her, she can lean back against the wall and wrap her legs around your waist as you enter her. Or, depending on the size of your shower/tub, you may be able to lie down and have her get on top and ride you as the water rushes over your bodies.

This One's for the Ladies

More often than not, quickies result in an orgasm . . . for him. Which is not to say she doesn't enjoy them too, but let's be honest, it's hard to come when you're pinned against a shower stall, right girls? Make this quickie for her. Once you're inside her, circle a bullet vibrator around her clitoris until she gets close to orgasm. Tell her to signal when she's about to come: She can squeeze your butt, bite your shoulder, sing the national anthem, whatever works for her. As she's climaxing, start thrusting through her orgasm until you come too (or not—remember, this one's for her).

Quick Tip:
Hang On

If shower sex is something you both love and want to make a regular activity, install a grab bar or two at strategic positions so you've got something to hang on to. You can also buy handles with super-strong suction cups and steps that attach to your shower walls specifically for this purpose. Google "sex in the shower products."

Quickie Bingo

Sit down together and dream up a list of possible quickie locations and scenarios. Don't limit yourselves to possibilities at home; also consider ideas out in the world (see "Playbook H: Quickie Locations" on page 167 for ideas). On a piece of blank paper or cardboard, draw a grid that looks like a bingo card. Enter your quickies from the list in each square and start working to fill up the card. When you fill out a line, celebrate with a longie. Full card? Start a new one!

One Hour or Less
Revising the Script

Often, when you've been together for a while, sex tends to follow a certain script. In most cases, it's the same script we've all followed since high school. Kissing, boobs, hands on each other's junk, maybe some oral and finally penetration. Change it up by writing some new scripts. Each of you writes down a bunch of things you enjoy sexually. They don't have to be fancy. It could be a certain position. It could be the order in which things happen. It could be that you enjoy five minutes of kissing instead of two. It could be where you have sex (see "Playbook H: Quickie Locations" on page 167 and "Playbook I: Field Trips" on pages 168–69 for ideas). Write them all down and keep these in your bedside drawers. Before you have sex, pick out a few items from each of your lists to come up with a fresh script for today's episode.

Quick Tip:
Mirror Image

Place a full-length mirror against the wall beside the bed so you can catch a reflection of the action. The excitement of watching yourselves will add to the heat.

Slide on In

Instead of him penetrating your vagina, squeeze some lube between your breasts, press them together and have him slide his erect penis between them. Tilt your head down and swirl your tongue around the tip as it emerges. Help him find some other fun places to park his pecker. For example, position yourself so he can glide his well-lubed penis back and forth between your butt cheeks, or slide his lubricated penis into other nooks and crannies, like your armpit or underneath your bent knee. See if he can get himself to orgasm by sliding his penis between the bottoms of your feet.

Slip 'n' Dip

Don't have time for a candlelit full-body massage? Get naked and tell him to lie back on the bed (throw some old towels or an old bedspread underneath to protect your sheets). Watch his eyes widen as you straddle his hips and proceed to drip oil onto his chest. Rub it across his pecs and around his nipples, using both hands. Wrap your oiled hands around his bicep. Glide them down the entire length of his arm, pressing your thumbs into his muscles and squeezing out through his fingertips. Repeat with his other arm and then each leg, from the tops of his thighs all the way down and out the tips of his toes. Move back up and slip your hands under his buttocks and give them a quick, firm massage. Slide your hand (add more oil, if necessary) up and down the shaft of his penis until he is standing at attention.

Quick Tip:
Sex on the Go

Carrying a quickie travel pack will make you more inclined to go for it when you suddenly find yourselves with an opportunity. Put the following in a small zippered pouch in your purse:

- A travel-sized tube of lube
- Some condoms (even if you don't use them for birth control or STI protection, they can help keep things tidy)
- A small egg-shaped or finger vibrator
- Some wet wipes for cleanup

Squat over his penis with your feet flat on either side of his hips as you lower yourself to just below the tip of his penis. Give him a squeeze, pull up and repeat a few times before slowly sliding down the entire length of his penis and back up again. Go back to lowering yourself to just below the tip for several strokes, squeezing the tip with your vaginal opening as you do. When you think he can't take it anymore, fake like you're going to slide all the way down and stop short, teasing him with a few more shallow dips before lowering yourself all the way down. Continue the tease—alternating between shallow and full dips—until he is close to orgasm. Now, stick to steady, fast, deep dips up and down the entire length of his member until you make him come . . . or your hamstrings give out.

All Night
Make It a Longie

I know, I know, scheduling time for sex doesn't feel romantic or, well, sexy. You want it to happen spontaneously like it did at the beginning of your relationship, blah, blah, blah. As I explained at the beginning of the book, it wasn't as spontaneous back then as you all like to believe. When you weren't together, you made it a priority to figure out when you might next be able to get your hands on each other naked. Between the opportunities to have sex, you spent time thinking about the sex you had last time and what you might do next time. It may not have felt like planning, but it was. Well now, when things are more familiar and especially when the rest of life gets in the way, you have to make a more conscious effort to make time for sex. And I mean quality sex.

Quickies are great, a furtive hand job in the movie theatre will certainly keep you lusting after one another, and sexy gestures every day will keep the spark alive on an ongoing basis, but every so often—whether

---

Quick Tip: Shifting Positions

Good intercourse isn't necessarily about twisting yourself into fancy positions (it's hard to focus on pleasure and just having fun if you're worried about whether your foot is caught in her armpit), but if you're looking to change things up, a different position can add variety, create new sensations for both parties and provide better access to certain body parts. Keep in mind that certain positions may get uncomfortable for one or both of you after a while. Be conscious of this and check in with each other regularly to make sure nothing's cramping or falling asleep. Depending on your height difference, certain positions will work better than others. Consult "Playbook J: Getting into Position" on pages 170–77 for inspiration.

twice a week or twice a month—you need a sex night. And if it's not happening naturally, you need to schedule. When you know a sex night (or morning or afternoon) is on the schedule, you'll be thinking about it beforehand and, when you get into the habit of it, you'll begin to anticipate these occasions with great excitement, maybe even thinking about something new you'd like to try or shopping for something sexy to wear. Then, with the luxury of more time, you can take things slowly, spend time wowing each other with all the great foreplay moves you've learned and, as I am about to show you, you can inject some interest into your intercourse. That doesn't sound so unromantic and unsexy, does it? All right then, just as you did to plan date nights back in the "Seduction" chapter, I want you to sit down with your devices right now and book your next sex date. Good.

Quick Tip:
Hot Lips

Before he even enters you, grab his erect penis and slide the tip up and down between your vaginal lips. He'll love the feeling of you taking control combined with the heavenly sensation of having the tip of his penis slide between your wet labia.

I've already given you plenty of material on how to make the getting naked and foreplay part of this sex date more exciting, so now I'd like to skip ahead to that glorious, breathtaking moment when you first enter her and see where we can go with this. Actually, let's step back a moment. Before you, um, take the plunge, let's drag this out and make her squirm a little, shall we?

Holding the shaft of your penis, push the tip in between her warm, wet labia and slide it up and down. Still holding on, run the now naturally lubricated tip of your penis back and forth across her clitoris and then in circles around it. She'll love to feel the firm but soft, wet tip against this sensitive spot. Tease her some more by dipping just the head of your penis into the opening of her vagina once or twice, then, when she's sufficiently out of her mind, slip just inside, pause for a second or two to look deep into her eyes and plunge deep. Hold off on thrusting for a moment. Stop and savour the feeling as you both melt into the connection, making direct eye contact for several seconds to help you both really focus on being in the moment. It seems simple, I know, so you may be surprised to discover that it's actually difficult, even uncomfortable, to look directly into your partner's eyes and hold their gaze during sex. That's what makes it so intense and wonderful. In that one moment, without saying a word, you can speak volumes to each other. You're telling each other, "I'm present, I see you, and nothing else exists but you and me in this moment. Where can we take it?"

Keep her guessing by adding some variety to your thrusts. For example, follow several quick shallow thrusts with a few slow deep thrusts, and then go back to quick and shallow. Okay, now try this: One slow shallow thrust, pause, two shallow thrusts, pause, three shallow thrusts, pause, and then bam, three quick deep thrusts. Hmmm, mmm.

Rather than stick to an in-and-out motion, get your whole pelvic area into it with some slooow rhythmic grinding (as opposed to painful mashing) and swivelling. Slide your penis deep inside her and swivel your hips as you grind them against her. Hold still for several seconds, letting her savour you deep inside her before you pull out and let just the tip of your penis push gently at the opening for another agonizing second or three. Then slide all the way in for several deep fast thrusts. Grab her hips with both hands and pull her toward you with a look that says "Hey hot stuff, I want those sexy hips closer to me so we can be even more connected and I can feel myself deeper inside you" without uttering a word.

Just a word of warning here: Changing things up when it comes to your thrusts is good, but you don't want to be switching things up so much that she thinks you've got attention deficit disorder. Think of it as a dance. You're leading but you're also responding to her body and the way she moves so that you can find the rhythm together.

Quick Tip:
Penetrating Thoughts

- Shallow thrusts stimulate the opening of her vaginal canal, which is crammed with nerve endings.
- Deep penetration gives her a sense of fullness and a strong sense of physical connection.
- Depending on how your bodies line up, deep thrusting may cause your pubic bone to bump into her clitoris and, in some cases, get her to orgasm during penetration.
- Depending on your size and hers, deep penetration may be painful for her. If this is a problem, circle your hand around the base of your penis to keep your thrusts shallow.

Besides driving up her excitement, keeping your thrusting varied and unpredictable gives you occasion to pause and regroup. This is helpful if a steady diet of fast deep thrusting has you coming before you want to. If you feel yourself close to orgasm (and haven't tipped over the "I have to come now" point of no return) but don't want to come, stop thrusting and stay still until the feeling of inevitable orgasm subsides. Then slowly start thrusting again and repeat. If you keep practising this cycle, you'll learn to have more control over when you come.

Don't ignore the rest of her. With your penis deep inside of her, pause and focus on really kissing her for a few minutes. Start with soft brushes of your tongue across her lips and neck. Gently tug her lower lip with your teeth. Run your tongue around her lips and slip it into her mouth, sliding it across her teeth before kissing her fully with soft but firm lips. Whisper something sexy in her ear, like how great it feels to be deep inside of her. Make it as PG or X-rated as you're comfortable with.

Stop thrusting for a minute and run your hands lightly around the sides of her breasts. Brush the back of your hand across her nipple. Alternate this with a firm, quick squeeze to vary the sensations. Run your fingers across the cheeks of her bum and let your fingernails graze the crease where it meets the tops of her legs. Light scratches, gentle caresses, light smacks and simple squeezes of bums, backs, thighs and shoulders keeps things surprising and exciting while providing a wonderful mix of feelings and stimulation.

On these wonderful occasions when you have more time for sex, take advantage of the opportunity to get creative. It's not important that you like everything you try when you experiment, but it *is* important that you like trying. Going in with an open mind is the best way to figure out what you like and don't like. Hopefully, you come out of it with a new trick or two that you can incorporate into your lovemaking on a regular basis. Experimentation is the best way to keep sex fresh, new and exciting.

Quick Tip:
Sounding It Out

There is something about the primal nature of sex that can bring out the inner potty mouth of even the most proper man or woman. Which can be hot. Even if you're uncomfortable with or turned off by explicit dirty talk, you can still be vocal. If you can't bring yourself to use actual words, use sound. Simply letting out a deep groan as you slide your penis inside her lets her know that she's turning you on, which in turn will, well, turn her on. Just make sure it's genuine. Fake or contrived moans, groans or dirty talk will achieve the opposite and turn your partner off.

You've test-driven some new thrusting styles, so now let's test-drive some toys. Toys can add a whole new level of pleasure to intercourse for both of you. If she has trouble reaching orgasm through penetration alone, using a vibrator on her clitoris while you're doing the old bump 'n' grind can help her get there. And, as I explained in the All Night section of "Hand Job for Him," vibrators can also add extra pleasure for you. There is also a whole crop of toys designed specifically for intercourse and, because the couples' market has exploded in recent years, the quality of toys just keeps getting better and better. Newer toys like the We-Vibe, for example, are designed to be worn during intercourse, so that one part of the vibe lies over her clitoris while the other part is inside her vagina, leaving enough room for your penis. When you slide inside, your penis pushes the vibe up against her G spot and you both feel the vibration.

Vibrating rings are one of many types of toys designed specifically to be used during intercourse. These are rubber, latex or silicone rings that have a tiny vibrator attached to them. You wear one around the base of your johnson and position it so that the wee vibrator makes contact with her baby johnson during penetration. Wearable vibrators have elastic straps that go around her hips and thighs so that the actual vibrator (usually in the shape of a butterfly or some other cutesy animal for some reason) sits over her clitoral area and can be worn during penetration. These types of vibrators will certainly add some sexy tingle to your tango, but if you want a toy that will get her to orgasm during intercourse, you'll

want to hit the target with a little more precision. Finger vibrators are great for this. They are worn—surprise—on your finger, making them easy to manoeuvre between your bodies and hold against her clitoris while all that writhing is going on. She can also cup a tiny egg- or bullet-shaped vibrator in her fingers and hold it against her clitoris during penetration. These tend to pack a bit more of a punch than finger vibes, perfect if your lady likes a more brawny buzz (every woman is different in terms of how much vibration she enjoys).

> ❝On these wonderful occasions when you have more time for sex, take advantage of the opportunity to get creative. It's not important that you like everything you try when you experiment, but it is important that you like trying.❞

Ultimately, any vibrating toy that one of you can manage to introduce to her little man in the canoe during intercourse will do the trick. Trying a few is the only way you'll find out what works for the two of you. Whichever toy you use, add some water- or silicone-based lube (note that silicone lube can't be used with silicone toys) to make things more comfy and deliciously slick. Depending on your vibe operating/thrusting coordination skills, you both might find it easier if she operates the machinery once you are inside so you can focus on your newly honed thrusting skills and she can control the intensity and directness of the vibration. (Ladies, if you're manning—or womanning, I guess—the controls as he thrusts, move the vibe around on your clitoris to see what feels good.) By the way, stud boy, be aware that she may find it challenging to hold the vibrator steady while you're doing all that creative hip work I taught you. Help her keep up. Slow down every five thrusts or so (something you should be doing anyway, young man, if you were paying attention earlier in this section). Stop thrusting completely every minute or so and plant some deep kisses on her mouth or breasts as she finds her rhythm. As her arousal ramps up you can start thrusting again, pausing or slowing down every so often to allow her to catch up before you go back to thrusting. This will improve your chances of reaching orgasm at, or close to, the same time, which can be incredibly intense.

Her orgasm shouldn't be the sole reason you use vibrators during sex. They are called toys for a reason. Use them to play. You can use a vibrator on her nipples or along the underside of her breasts. She can run a vibrator along the sensitive underside of your erection and around the tip before you enter her, or tickle your testicles or nipples with one during intercourse.

> 66 Stop thrusting completely every minute or so and plant some deep kisses on her mouth or breasts as she finds her rhythm. 99

Using a vibrator is one way for her to achieve orgasm during intercourse. But it's not the only way. Whenever you've got some extra time to play, use it to test-drive some of the different ways you can make each other come. Ladies, you don't necessarily need a vibrator to pay attention to your clitoris during intercourse. Fingers work too. If you're in the missionary position with him on top and you on your back, wiggle your hand down between your bodies you so you can play with your clitoris. If you usually masturbate lying on your back (see, this is where that masturbating practice pays off), this will feel familiar and you can use the same moves. Only here, you get the added pleasure of feeling him inside you while you do.

Any position (see "Playbook J: Getting into Position" on pages 170–77 for more details) that allows you to reach down and play will work, of course. If you're doing it doggie-style, try supporting yourself on one arm or elbow while you use the other hand to reach down and stimulate your clitoris. If you're lying on your side with him lying on his side behind you, you can reach down between your legs while he enters you.

Quick Tip:
First-Come Basis
If you're worried about lasting during intercourse, bring her to orgasm orally or manually before you enter the pearly gates and she'll be less concerned about how long you spend inside.

Then again, how amazing would it be to feel his hands on your tender bits as he's sliding in and out of you? While you're doing it doggie-style he can reach around your hips and get his hands up in your business. If you both kneel upright on the bed, with you in front, he can lean back to rest his bum on his heels as you lower yourself onto him, and he can reach around and play with you with his fingers. Try some other positions to see what kind of fun trouble you can get yourselves into.

Your best chance at achieving a G-spot orgasm through intercourse is to try a position that will angle his penis so that it rides along the front inside wall of your vagina. Some penises are conveniently curved upward so that this happens in the missionary position. If your guy's not particularly curvy, entering you from behind will put his penis in line with the target. Girl on top also works nicely for this purpose. Play around and see what works for the two of you. You'll know you've hit the spot when, after a minute or two of him sliding back and forth across the area, you start to feel pressure or a feeling almost like you have to pee. You may even feel the urge to push. If you went to the bathroom before sex, you can be confident that your bladder is empty and go with the urge. Bear down (pushing on your pubic bone with your hand as you do so can help) while he continues to thrust. Keep at it and you may eventually feel a sense of release during which you may expel a small—or sometimes a large—amount of clear liquid from your vagina. Congratulations! You've just had a G-spot orgasm. If it doesn't happen, don't sweat it. Despite the hype, a G-spot orgasm is not necessarily better than a clitoral orgasm, just different. Not every woman can or necessarily wants to experience one. If you do want to, well, you'll just have to schedule some more quality sex time so you can keep trying.

Quick Tip:
Direct Action

Sometimes, all it takes is a well-timed hip wiggle or moan to communicate what you like (or don't like) during sex. Other times, getting what you want in bed requires more direct communication. You want to offer suggestions, but you hold off. You're shy or you don't want to say the wrong thing. Meanwhile, your brain is constructing a full seminar and workshop on how to make you come and you end up so distracted by your own self-conscious thoughts that you start to lose it. You try to relax, grit your teeth and focus while chanting inside your head, "I will have an orgasm, I will have an orgasm." Not so productive. Sure, it's lovely when he can read your body's response and intuit your needs, but no one is a mind reader. Having to ask for something sexually doesn't make it less valuable or mean that he cares any less. It just means he doesn't know everything you like at all times and at every stage in your sexual life. So, yes, you have to tell him.

There are things you can do to enhance his climax as well. For example, as he's getting close to orgasm, squeeze your vagina with each thrust so he feels you tighten around his penis. Open up and invite him in by pushing out as he's entering, then pull your vaginal muscles in nice and tight as he's pulling out, kind of like your vagina is giving him a hand job. Continue to do this until he comes. Then pulse your PC muscles a few times as he orgasms to complete the job. Alternatively, while he's inside of you, circle your thumb and forefinger around the base of his penis. As he pulls out, let the shaft slide through the snug finger circle you've created. Turn it into a "canal" by adding the other fingers. As he thrusts in and out of your extended love canal, it will feel like he's getting a hand job and having intercourse at the same time—sure to send him over the edge. I know he adores the sensation of coming inside you. But next time you feel him getting close to orgasm, ask him to pull out so you can take him in your mouth and bring him to orgasm that way. I guarantee he won't complain.

Every couple loves the idea of coming together. Releasing all that oxytocin (the bonding hormone that is secreted by both men and women during orgasm) at the same time makes you feel connected and close. In the movies and in porn, couples magically erupt into simultaneous orgasm every time they have sex, seemingly with little effort on anyone's part. We've seen this model for so long, it's hard not to believe this is how it should happen every time in real life. It rarely does. Luckily, there are ways to enjoy coming simultaneously or at least close together during intercourse that don't require any acting skills:

Quick Tip: Don't Be Too Hard on Yourself

While most men have a much greater guarantee of orgasm through intercourse than women do, some guys have a hard time coming this way. If this happens to him, most likely his instinct is to start thrusting harder and faster, thinking this will make him come. Ironically, hard thrusting usually succeeds in further desensitizing his penis. In this case, he may need additional stimulation from you. Maybe he likes to have his nipples pinched, or his testicles gently tugged, or the back of his neck nibbled. Also, nobody says a legitimate orgasm has to happen inside you. If he wants to come and it's not happening through penetration, ask him to pull out so you can stimulate him manually or orally. Or ask him to put on a show for you and masturbate himself to orgasm.

• Masturbate to the brink of orgasm and, as you are both getting close (you might want to establish a signal or bring a small flag to bed to wave at the exact moment you're ready), have him enter you and, with a few thrusts of his magic penis, if you get the timing just right, you'll both tumble over the brink together.

• Use a vibrator on yourself while he watches and strokes himself almost to orgasm. Have him enter you as you both climax.

• Have him go down on you while he strokes himself, being careful not to come. When you're both getting close and waving your flags (though he may have his hands full, so he could just growl "Now, baby" or something) go penis to vagina and hope you're both winners in your little game of Catch My Orgasm If You Can.

> **There are ways to enjoy coming simultaneously or at least close together during intercourse that don't require any acting skills.**

However your session ends, take a few minutes to bask in those blissful after-sex moments when you're both lying there, bodies entangled, drooling slightly, and everything looks kind of blurry—before one of you finally gets up to grab something from the laundry hamper to clean up the mess. Take advantage of this wonderful time to experience your connection and the heightened sense of intimacy you're no doubt both feeling. He may not want to call it cuddling, but I doubt he'd turn down a few extra moments of feeling your soft, naked body curled up against him after the act. Despite the grief guys get for dozing off after sex, falling asleep together can be perfectly desirable and lovely for both parties. Especially if it's late and you both have an early morning. It also depends on the intensity of your orgasm. If it's one of those that leaves your legs rubbery and your ability to speak impaired, some quiet spooning time is definitely required—until a limb falls asleep and you roll over, curl into fetal positions and pass out.

If neither of you is sleepy, life's been crazy and you've been feeling a bit like two ships in the night, this quiet, intimate time is a great opportunity for some "Hey, I know you. What have you been up to?" catch-up. Also, fantasies may not seem like the most obvious thing to discuss, but the pleasant lull after sex can be a great time to explore—to talk about what you'd like to try. You're feeling open and intimate and, since you've just had sex, there's no pressure to do anything about it right away (at least not if you don't want to). Use this time to build some sexual anticipation and give your partner something to savour until you have sex again. Describe something you liked about what just transpired and maybe add a new twist you might like to give it in the future. And just like that, afterplay becomes foreplay for the next time you have sex.

> ❝After sex can be a great time to explore fantasies—to talk about what you'd like to try.❞

Quick Tip: Wake-up Call

If your guy is a notorious post-coital snoozer, he's not necessarily being insensitive or uncaring. His chemical makeup may be to blame. After orgasm, both men and women enter the "resolution phase" of the sexual response cycle. The problem is, men nosedive through this phase in about a minute, while women enjoy a more gentle descent, taking about five or ten minutes to come down. If you want to discourage him from nodding off, tell him that maintaining physical contact after orgasm is an important step in becoming a multi-orgasmic male. Ask him to stay inside of you instead of withdrawing after his orgasm as you continue to caress and kiss (this is not recommended if you're wearing a condom, of course). Chances are, his need to relax or sleep will recede behind a surge of growing arousal that will make him want to start all over again.

PLAYBOOK H
QUICKIE LOCATIONS

CARS

Cars are great for quickies because you can park them wherever you want. Heck, go have a quickie in the car in the garage right now. If you want the added thrill of knowing someone could walk by at any time, climb onto his lap in the front seat while you're in a parking lot. If you want more privacy, find a dead-end road or cul-de-sac.

CLOSETS

Pretend you're at a high-school party and sneak off to neck in the closet. Only now you don't have to be concerned about how many bases you're going to steal. She'll let you get all the way to home plate.

PICNICS

Wear your most full, flouncy skirt, pack a picnic and head to the park. Find a quiet, secluded spot behind a tree or two and lay your blanket on the ground. After you've shared some wine and fed each other grapes, climb onto his lap, pull your panties to one side and spread out your skirt to hide the show.

FITTING ROOMS

She slips in to try something on and, when the salesclerk isn't looking, you slip in after her and she tries you on instead. If there's a bench, she can prop one leg on it and hang on to the top of the dressing room wall for extra support.

PUBLIC WASHROOMS

Given today's climate of extreme germ phobia, I fear this quickie classic is losing its appeal for many. But you can't underestimate the excitement of returning to your table to rejoin friends at a bar or restaurant knowing your sweetie just did you pinned up against the bathroom stall wall.

AT HOME

While you're both at work and the kids are at school, arrange to meet for "lunch." Go home and enjoy a quickie in the comfort of your very own bed before heading back to the office.

PLAYBOOK I
FIELD TRIPS

There is absolutely nothing wrong with having sex in bed. In fact, after spending your formative years finding locations to have sex where you wouldn't get caught by your parents (cars, closets, bathroom stalls or wherever kids sneak off to), it's rather nice as an adult to have sex in the comfort of your grown-up, four-hundred-thread-count Egyptian cotton sheets. But when you're busy, overworked and exhausted, it's often more tempting to fall asleep in the bed than have sex in it. You're far less likely to fall asleep when you're doing it on the kitchen table. Something as simple as changing where you have sex can really turn up the sexual heat. That's why vacation sex is often hotter than at-home sex. The change of scenery takes you out of your comfort zone and allows you to see each other against a different backdrop. But you don't need an exotic location or an expensive resort. The beauty of this simple trick is that it doesn't have to take any more time than it does to walk from your bedroom to your living room.

SEX AROUND THE HOUSE
The kitchen table (just remove sharp objects and clean up afterward; people have to eat off of that thing), the couch or living room rug, the laundry room (where there are usually lots of dirty towels around for cleanup afterward), the kids' room (okay, maybe not)—all are great potential sex locations. (Though unless you want your kids to walk in on the two of you doing it in their toy room, you might want to make sure they're not going to be coming home in the next ten minutes or so.)

SLY SEX
The idea of potentially getting caught can create urgency and excitement whether you're having full intercourse in the bathroom at a party (just be quick, others have to pee) or copping a feel under the table while you're out to dinner with friends. Trying to pretend nothing's going on is not only playful and deliciously naughty, it forces you to react differently to familiar sensations, making them feel brand spanking new. Trying to have quiet sex while houseguests are sleeping (or possibly having hot, quiet sex too) in the next room is also a great way to achieve this feeling. Ditto when you're a guest somewhere. (Though, unlike in a hotel, you need to remember to clean up after yourselves.)

HOTEL SEX

Having sex in a hotel allows you to get away from your home environment and its usual distractions and responsibilities. And who says you have to travel anywhere to stay in a hotel? Search discount websites and find a cheap rate for a local hotel, pack an overnight bag and check in. Order room service and spend the night together. No watching TV or passing out.

OUTDOOR SEX

Barring insects, sunburn in places where the sun doesn't usually shine, wildlife and human intrusions, sex in the great outdoors is a fine way to feel at one with nature. Feeling the sun hitting your naked bodies on a blanket in the middle of a field, or the evening breeze under the stars on a warm summer night is exhilarating. Why do you think nudists are so keen on running around naked?

SEX IN WATER

If you're lucky enough to have a tub big enough for two (it's hard to feel sexy with your knees wedged into your eye sockets), baths can be a great place to get intimate. Have her sit between your legs facing forward so she can lie back against your chest. In this position, you can give her breasts and shoulders a nice soapy sponge-down. If you've got a removable shower head (or a waterproof sex toy), you can use it to get her off while she lies back comfortably (see "Bathing Beauty" on page 81). Switch positions and she's in a perfect spot to give you a nice wet, slippery hand job.

SEX IN MOTION

Having sex in the bathroom of a train or a plane is tempting, though it's challenging enough doing your business in one of those things—coordinating two adult bodies into any kind of sexual position has injury written all over it. But the thrill may be worth the challenge and the risk. Just be sure to put the toilet seat down first. You don't want spillage.

PLAYBOOK J
GETTING INTO POSITION

According to whoever takes the time to count these things, there are an estimated six hundred sex positions out there for the trying. Don't have time to try them all? Not to worry: Most are variants of the following six basic positions. Surely you can find the time to try all six at least once over the next few weeks, months or year. Once you get the basics down, you're only as limited as your flexibility.

MISSIONARY

A true classic that never goes out of style. Sure, it sounds a little pious, but there's something deliciously naughty about its religious connotations. Plus, it's relatively comfortable (though slightly more physically demanding for him), doesn't require advanced gymnastic skills and lets you have intercourse face to face, allowing for lots of kissing and eye contact. Yum.

How to do it: She lies on her back with her legs spread apart, knees bent and feet flat on the bed. He positions himself over her, lying face down with his legs between hers, supporting his lower body on his bent knees and supporting his upper body with his arms as he penetrates her.

Take It Up a Notch
Her
- Stimulate your clitoris with your hands or a vibrator while he is penetrating you.
- Grab his bum with your hands and control his thrusts.

Him
- Pin her hands over her head to exercise a little playful dominance (just be sure to let her go if she wants to use her hands to get in on the action below).
- If you have a lot of upper-body strength, lower yourself down on your arms to kiss her mouth or breasts.

Variations
- She wraps her legs around his bum—this will allow her to control the pace and depth of his thrusts.

- She places her legs inside his and closes her thighs nice and tight. This limits the depth of his penetration but can still feel great for him as his penis slides between her closed thighs and into her vagina.

- Depending on her flexibility, she stretches one leg straight out on the bed and raises the other in the air. He kneels with one knee on either side of her lower leg and penetrates her while holding on to her raised leg for support. Heck, raise both legs up if you can muster it (oh, and congratulations, by the way).

- She pulls her knees up tight to her chest with her feet in the air. He kneels in front of her, leaning his torso against the back of her thighs. She can rock back and forth to meet his thrusts.

- Place pillows underneath her bum to raise her pelvis and change the angle of penetration. He can also do this by sliding his hands underneath her hips and raising her bum as he penetrates her.

DOGGIE-STYLE

Or, if you prefer, *position de la levrette,* as the French call it (*levrette* means "greyhound," as in dog not bus). This position doesn't allow for much eye contact or kissing but he does get a sweet view of her bottom as he enters her. This angle directs the penis along the inside front wall of her vagina, allowing for potential G-spot stimulation.

How to do it: She is on all fours with her knees and hands spread for support while he kneels behind her so that he can penetrate her from this position. Place a pillow under his knees for comfort.

Take It Up a Notch
Her

- While he's thrusting, slide your hand down your stomach to stimulate your clitoris with your fingers or a vibrator.

Him

- While you're penetrating her from behind, reach around to stimulate her clitoris with your fingers or a vibrator.

Variations

- She lowers her upper body to support herself on her forearms instead of her hands. This raises her bum higher in the air and allows for deeper penetration.
- She lies flat on her tummy. Penetration isn't as deep, but he gets the added stimulation of feeling his penis glide between her thighs and butt cheeks as he slides in and out.

SIDE BY SIDE

Also referred to as spooning, this sweet, intimate and comfortable position allows for lots of close body contact and touching.

How to do it: Both of you lie on your sides facing the same direction so that her back is against his chest and her bum is nestled into his crotch. That's right, just like spooning, but with penetration. He slides his penis between her thighs and enters her from behind as she pushes her bum back into him. Depending on your heights, you may need to shift your bodies up or down to achieve the right angle.

Take It Up a Notch

Her

- Reach down between your legs and give yourself a hand as he penetrates you.
- Reach back to caress and squeeze his butt and control his thrusting.

Him

- Reach around to her front to stroke her breasts and play with her clitoris.

Variations

- Changing the position of her legs will vary the angle and depth of penetration. She can swing her top leg forward and tilt her pelvis down toward the bed or pull both knees up to her chest. He shifts his entire body down to achieve a good position for penetration.
- She lies facing him with her top leg bent over his hip. He may need to shift his body down to achieve the right angle for penetration. Deep penetration may not be possible, but this position allows for lots of kissing, fondling and eye contact.

HER ON TOP

Also known as the cowgirl, as in "Ride him, cowgirl!" Most women like this position because it allows them to control the pace and depth of his thrusting. He'll love it because he gets to lie back comfortably and get a great view.

How to do it: She sits on top of him with her legs on either side of him, knees bent and shins on the bed. In this position, she can lower herself down and raise herself up on his penis.

Take It Up a Notch

Her

- Lean back, bracing yourself with your arms. Use your legs to push yourself up as he watches his penis slide out of your vagina. Stop before it slides out completely and pause, holding the tip of his penis just inside your vagina. Look into his eyes and smile before slowly sliding all the way back down.
- Grind your pelvis into his, rubbing your clitoris against his pubic bone.
- Reach down and stimulate your clitoris with your fingers or a vibrator. Make a show of playing with your breasts. Lean over and graze your nipples against his.

Variations

- Instead of her resting on her knees and shins, she can squat with her feet flat on the bed. This gives her even more control because she can use her legs to push as she slides her body up and down his penis.
- She turns around so her back is facing him in a position often referred to as the reverse cowgirl. She leans backward, lowering her back to his chest to create a more natural angle for his penis to enter her. Leaning back in the reverse cowgirl also makes it easy to reach down to her clitoris.
- While in the reverse cowgirl, she leans forward, bracing her upper body with her arms. This way he gets a great view of her bum and his penis entering her vagina. Just be careful not to bend his penis too far in the wrong direction.
- He lies back on the bed with his bum positioned right at the edge and his legs hanging over, feet flat on the floor. She stands over him, straddling his legs, feet flat on the floor, and lowers herself onto his penis. Pressing his feet into the floor, he pushes his pelvis up to meet her thrusts as she rides his penis. She can lean forward on her elbows for more stability and control.

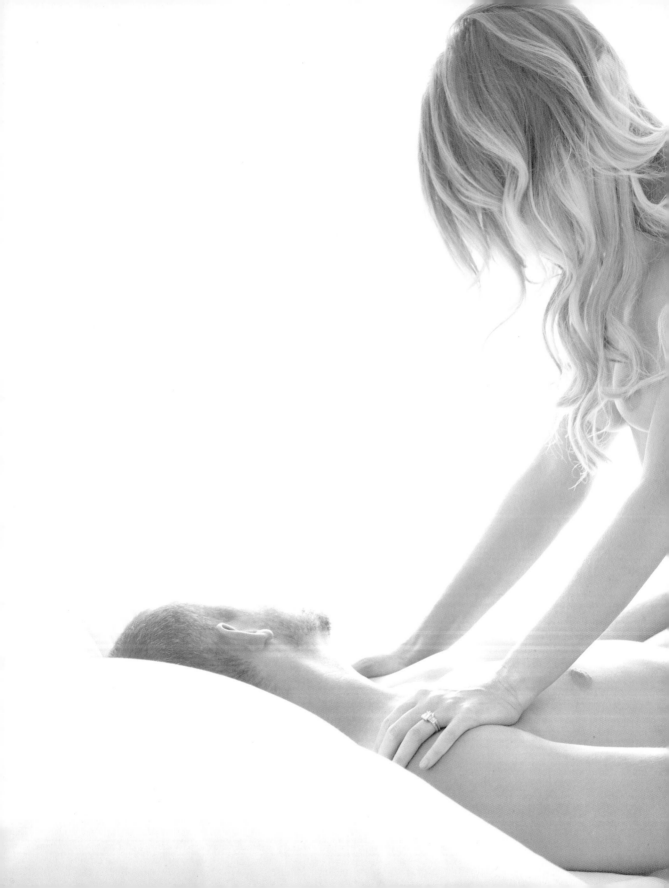

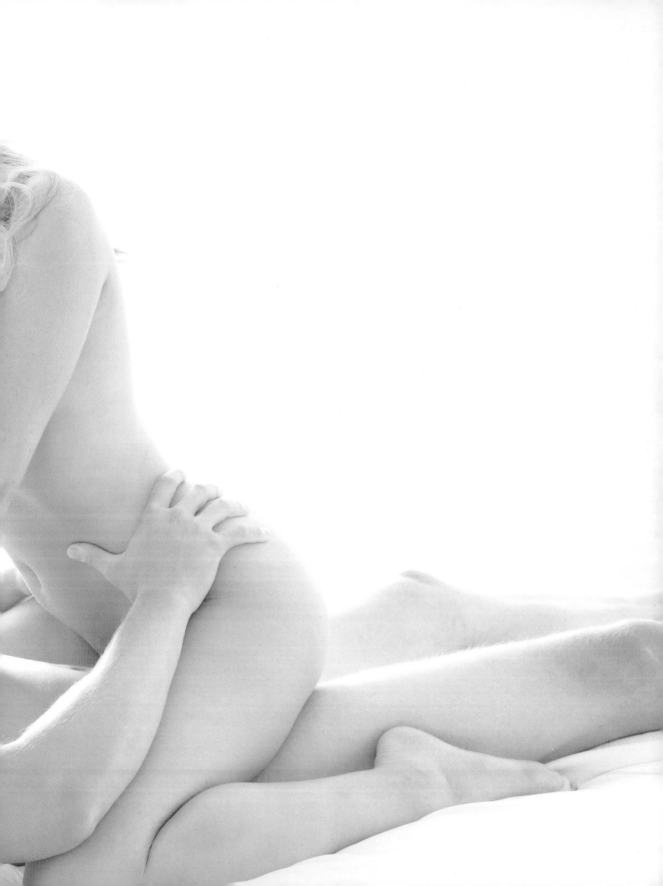

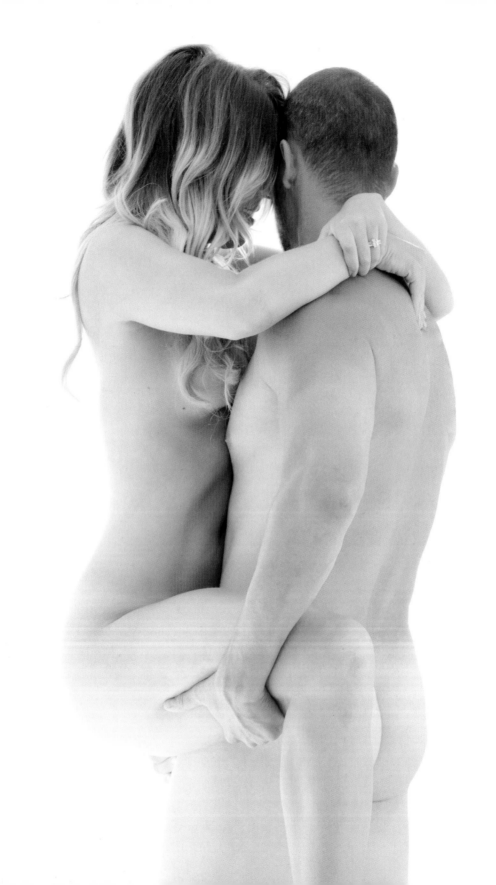

STANDING

Because they require quite a lot of stamina, especially on his part, standing positions aren't recommended for all-night lovemaking sessions (which is not to say you can't toss some stand-up sex into the evening's mix). But because having sex standing up doesn't require wasting any time on silly things like finding a bed or lying down, it can be a great position for quickies.

How to do it: Depending on the difference in your heights, trying to have face-to-face sex with both of you actually standing up can be awkward. She can sit on the edge of a table, washing machine, deck railing (be careful of splinters!), countertop (be sure to wipe up any crumbs) or anything that puts her at hip level, while he stands in front of her between her legs.

Take It Up a Notch

Her

- Wrap your legs around his bum so you can grind into him and control his thrusting by using your calves to pull his butt toward you.

Him

- Deepen penetration (and get a great view of your penis entering her) by holding up one of her legs with one arm while you penetrate her.

Variations

- She bends over at the waist so he can enter her from behind. She can brace herself against a wall or lean forward over a table or bench for support so she can grind her bum back into his pelvis.
- He can impress her with his strength. As she leans back against a wall, facing him, he lifts her legs up with both arms and wraps them around his hips, pressing her back into the wall to help support her weight as he penetrates her.

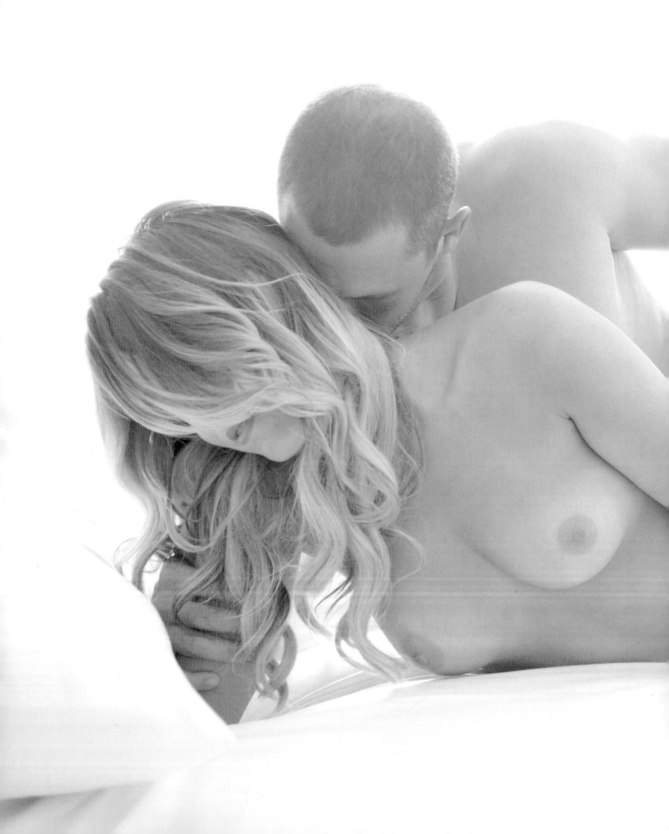

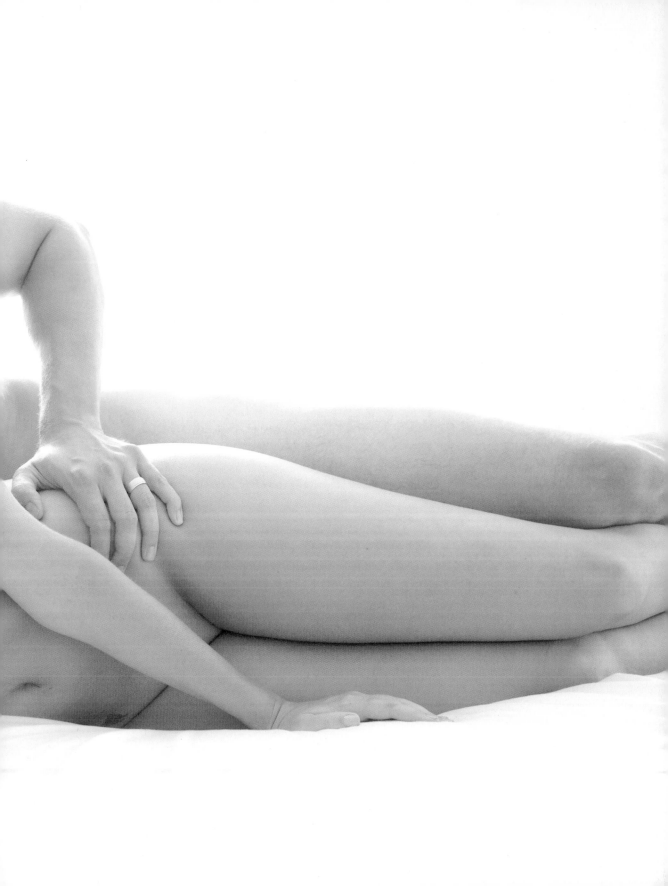

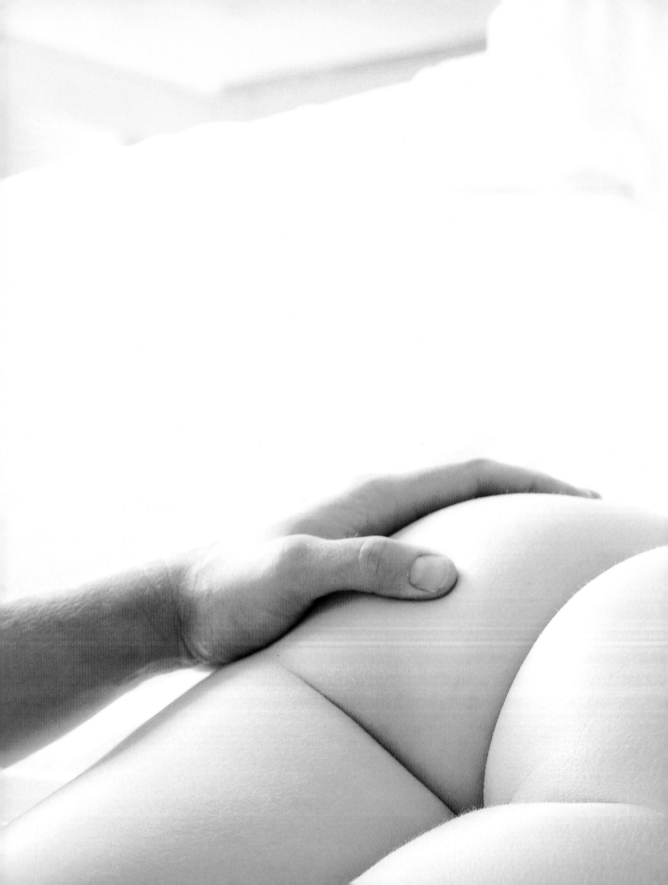

Chapter Eleven
ANAL

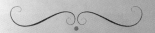

I suspect that even if the two of you haven't gone there, or even talked about it, one—or both—of you has been just a little bit curious about anal sex. I don't blame you. Just as talking about or, heaven forbid, engaging in oral sex pushed the sexual envelope for your parents or grandparents, anal sex seems to be the sexual frontier of today's generation. Some of the curiosity stems from its still somewhat culturally taboo quality. It makes you feel naughty. And because it involves one of the most private areas of your body, butt play is very intimate and can make you feel extremely vulnerable, which is both sexy and scary. That's why it requires plenty of trust, communication . . . and lube.

Anal play is probably not something you're going to explore every time you have sex, but, given that your derrière is home to a whole whack of wonderfully sensitive nerve endings and potential pleasure, it would be a shame to ignore it completely. And given that you're often down there doing other stuff anyway, it seems silly not to at least try stopping in. If you don't like it, no one says you have to make a return visit.

Obviously, I'm not going to recommend an anal sex bathroom stall quickie. Anal play is not something you rush, and you'll most likely want to save any elaborate bum play plans for occasions when you have more time. You can, however, add a quick anal twist to other sexual activities. Okay, maybe "twist" is the wrong word. When it comes to your tush, twisting is not recommended, especially for beginners.

I suggest you begin by talking about it. While certain sexual surprises are fun for her (a gift certificate for a half-hour session of receive-only oral sex springs to mind), anal sex is not one of them. Sure, there may be a time when things are hot and heavy and you're both feeling extremely turned on and brave enough to give anal sex a whirl. But if you haven't already discussed technique or boundaries, chances are it won't go very well, and the back door may be permanently closed to any future visits. If you've had a conversation or two beforehand and

then, in the heat of the moment, you both decide you're willing to go there, there's a much better chance of it being a hot, enjoyable experience that you'll want to try again.

I know that talking to each other about trying anything sexually new can be scary. What if he reacts negatively? What if she thinks you're a sexual freak? But being sexually curious is absolutely normal. And if you don't even talk to each other about your sexual wants and desires, your sex life is guaranteed to remain right where it is, in a holding pattern of predictability, eventual boredom and, most likely, disinterest. Surely, avoiding all that is worth a tiny bit of risk. At the very least, even if you don't end up trying anal sex, forcing yourself to explore the topic will get you talking about sex and help to improve your sexual communication in general.

If you don't know how to bring up the topic, you might find it easier to refer to something you saw or read. "Honey, I was reading this amusing article the other day about how anal sex is the new black and more and more couples are exploring anal play. Have you ever thought about it? I think it'd be kind of hot." If your partner's reaction is "Eew, that's gross!" remain open and try to find out what they find gross about it. If cleanliness is a concern, talk about how to deal with any potential mess: Shower beforehand, make sure you've gone to the bathroom and wear a latex glove during digital penetration, a condom during anal sex or a latex dental dam if you're using your mouth in the area. Your partner's resistance may be psychological. They may worry that, if they go along with this, you'll want to try other freaky stuff they might not be ready for. Assure them that you would never make them do something they didn't want to and that this is simply about wanting to explore something new and potentially fun together.

This is also your opportunity to negotiate boundaries. For example, if you've promised her you'll stop any attempt at penetration immediately if she asks, she will feel more relaxed, respected and trusting. He might be willing to have you explore the area without penetration, maybe just a well-lubricated finger rubbed around the area. Or if he isn't game for anal penetration with your finger or a toy, would he be open to feeling your tongue on his anus, perhaps with a latex dental dam covering it, if he's concerned about cleanliness?

On that note, I'd like to first dispel a few rumours about anal play:

• One of the first fears people have is that they might encounter fecal matter. Okay, not totally a rumour. With deeper penetration, you might, but honestly, it's unlikely. The anal canal is simply a passageway en route to the exit and not a storage vessel.

If you're concerned, like I said, go to the bathroom first.

• Many women who are curious but nervous about trying anal sex have asked me, "Does it honestly feel good?" I assure you, it can feel good, and yes, there are women who genuinely enjoy anal sex. Honest.

• Many women are afraid that anal play equals pain. Not if it's done right.

There are also a couple of safety precautions I'd like you to heed:

• Don't numb the area. Certain lubes marketed specifically for anal sex contain benzocaine or a similar anaesthetic that is meant to numb your bum to lessen potential pain. But pain is your signal that something's not right, and you don't want to dull such important feedback.

• Don't drink and have bum sex. Alcohol sometimes provides the liquid courage to try things you've been sexually curious about, so it's not uncommon for couples to attempt anal sex for the first time bolstered by a few drinks. While there's nothing wrong with having a glass of wine to relax, having too much to drink may lower your inhibitions to the point that you aren't careful and someone could get hurt.

The LAY of the LAND

Before we get started, you need to know what you're dealing with. When it comes to anal sex, the bum parts we're concerned with are the anal canal and the rectum. It varies from person to person, but the anal canal is about two inches long and is home to a couple of muscular rings known as the internal and external sphincters. (Whoever named all our bum bits was clearly not a fan of anal sex or they'd have made it all sound a lot sexier, but stick with me, this is important stuff if you plan on going there.) The external sphincter is your anus, or butt hole, if you prefer. Just inside a ways is the internal sphincter, the gateway to your rectum. You can tense and relax your anus voluntarily. Try it right now. Easy, right? But the internal sphincter is a bit trickier. It is controlled by your nervous system and less willing to relax on command. In fact, when someone or something tries to enter rather than exit, its natural tendency is to circle the troops and shut the gate. However, with some practice, breathing and patience, you can get the two sphincters to work as a team and convince them that what's happening is a good thing that you are in full agreement with.

Once you get past the internal sphincter, you enter the hallowed halls of your rectum, a tube about ten inches long that connects your colon to the anus. When it comes to anal play, the important thing about your rectum is that it's not a straight tube but a bit of a winding road. You'll have to keep your eyes—or more accurately, your fingers, toys or penis—on this road in order to make anal penetration comfortable.

TIME to PLAY

Five Minutes or Less

Share a Tail Tale

Email him a link to an erotic online story that includes anal play. In your note, ask him to send it back with his favourite bits highlighted.

Discover Each Other's Bottom Lines

Make a list of the reasons you do and don't want to try anal play. Include things you're curious about, afraid of, excited by. Share your lists over a glass of wine and use the opportunity to have an honest discussion about your feelings regarding anal play.

Slip into Your Seat

The next time you're in the shower alone, let your soapy, slippery finger do a little walking. A little self-exploration will familiarize you with the territory and help you wrap your head around the idea of having someone else pokin' around down there.

One Hour or Less

Explore the Surrounding Area

If you're curious about anal play but still feel hesitant, stick to the outlying regions. After all, bum play doesn't have to involve entry to be enjoyable. Get naked together and have her lie on her stomach as you start massaging, squeezing and tickling her buttocks. Trickle some lube between her cheeks and slide your entire hand sideways between them. If she seems to be enjoying herself, press the flat of your thumb against her anus and glide up and down or make circles around the opening. Slip several fingers of your other hand into her vagina, sliding them in and out, or see if you can wiggle your fingers up to her clitoris as you continue to massage her anus. If you have trouble bringing her to orgasm this way, ask her if she'd like to help. Continue playing with her bum —tickling her cheeks, massaging and circling her anus with your thumb — while she reaches down and masturbates herself to orgasm. Variation: If you're not ready to use toys for penetration, you can still have some anal fun with them. The area around your rectum is full of nerves and simply twirling a vibrator around this area is a great way to stimulate them.

Tactile Pleasure

In the "Hand Job for Him" section, I showed her how to use her fingers to stimulate the male G spot via your anus. She doesn't have a G spot in her bottom, but your fingers can still offer it much pleasure. Also, if the two of you are thinking you might eventually like to go all the way and enjoy anal intercourse, practising first with your fingers is a great idea. You'll get to know the territory intimately, and fingers offer better tactile feedback than your penis. This will also help her get used to the feeling of anal penetration with an object smaller, and therefore less intimidating, than your penis.

AT YOUR FINGERTIPS

Lube

Latex glove or finger cot

Before you start, make sure your nails are trimmed and filed. Anal tissue is thin and, well, ouch. You may want to wear a latex glove or a finger cot (like a little latex sock for your finger), both of which can be purchased at most pharmacies. Whether you're covering up or not, as with any type of anal play, always use plenty of water-based lube (especially if you're using latex, as anything oil-based will destroy the latex). By now you know to warm things up by kissing her, playing with her breasts and teasing her with touch. Now, have her lie on her tummy and spend time massaging, squeezing, tickling and kissing her butt cheeks. Run a hand down between her thighs and then run it sideways up between her buns.

Squeeze some lube onto your fingers and circle the flat pad of your index finger around the opening of her anus. Allow her to get used to the sensation. As she relaxes, press gently at the opening. Go back to circling. Make eye contact and give her a smile to see how she's doing. If she smiles back, you've got the thumbs-up. Press the pad of your finger more firmly against the opening until the tip slips inside. When you feel the resistance from the sphincter muscle, don't push. Stop, let her take a few deep breaths and, as you feel the muscle relax and draw you in, slowly glide your finger inside.

Once inside, try some slow, teasing strokes in and out. Twist your finger back and forth. Go back to stroking. Check in regularly to make sure everything is okay and that she wants you to continue. If she discovers that she enjoys having your finger in her bottom, you can incorporate it into other types of sex play. Having your finger in her bottom while you're going down on her, for example, will feel exquisite. And just imagine the pleasure you could bring her if you were to stimulate her clitoris, penetrate her vagina and slip a finger into her bottom all at the same time. Oh my.

Kissing Butt

Frankly, neither the term "analingus" nor the perhaps more familiar slang moniker "rimming" make this activity sound very sexy. It's no wonder so many people immediately go "ick" at the very thought of getting their tongue anywhere near their partner's bottom. If you haven't picked up on this already, there are lots of yummy nerve endings in and around the anus. And just as having a nice, warm, soft wet tongue caressing other sensitive parts of your body feels good, that same tongue tickling all the lovely nerve endings in and around your bum can feel wonderful. And the taboo nature of this activity adds a naughty "I can't believe we're doing this" adventurous aspect to sex.

You'll both feel more confident and relaxed if you know everything's squeaky clean. Have a shower beforehand, or hey, come to think of it, kneeling in the shower and sliding your tongue across your partner's bottom as the water rushes over your bodies would be pretty scorchin'.

If you're still squeamish about the idea of direct tongue-to-bum contact, cover the area with a latex dental dam, or cut the tip off a condom, slice it down the side and roll it flat. If neither of these is handy, cover the area with a piece of plastic wrap. This may not sound very sexy but, when your sweetheart's moaning with pleasure as you slide your warm, slippery, flat tongue across the plastic, you'll quickly change your mind.

The two most comfortable positions

for analingus are either to have your partner on all fours with you kneeling behind or to have your partner on their back with their knees pulled up to their chest and you lying on your belly just as if you were going to perform oral sex . . . only a little lower. In fact, an obvious time to explore his bum with your tongue is during fellatio, while your mouth is already down there, you've got him turned on and everything's already good and wet. Adding some tongue-to-bum action when you're going down on her is a little trickier because of the risk of transferring bacteria from the rectum to the delicate, thin tissue of her vagina. To avoid this, make sure her bum is nice and clean before you start and use a latex or plastic barrier.

Whether you make analingus an extension of oral sex or a treat all on its own, don't head straight for the target. If you're kneeling behind him, spend time caressing and planting light kisses across his bum. Run your finger between the cheeks, letting your fingernail lightly graze the skin, following this with a string of kisses along the crevice. Gently spread his buttocks with your hands and blow warm breath against his anus. Now slide a flat, wet tongue from the base of his testicles all the way to his tailbone, dragging your tongue across his anus en route. Point your tongue and swirl it around the opening. Every few circles around the rim, dart your tongue in and out a few times.

This is a great way to experiment with the sensation of anal penetration because the tongue is relatively short and soft, so there's no potential pain. You're unlikely to get your partner to orgasm through analingus alone, but you can certainly give him a hand job or have him masturbate to orgasm while your tongue is working its magic. And you, young man, could try some of the great moves you learned in the "Hand Job for Her" section to add some extra pleasure.

All Night

From Top to Bottom

So you've discovered you quite enjoy a little bum play and want to expand your horizons but are still a little nervous about going all the way. Start the evening by experimenting with some toys made specifically for anal play, like butt plugs and anal beads (see the "Toys" appendix for more detailed info). Any anal toy should be flared at the base (because you don't want to be losing anything up in there) and well lubed. Spend time warming his buns by massaging and kissing his bottom, massaging his thighs and running the toy up and down between his cheeks. As he gets excited, twirl the lubed toy around the opening of the anus to allow his bum to relax, open up and invite you in. Then very gently nudge the tip of the toy (or the first bead if you're using anal beads) into the opening and stop to let him relax and draw the toy in as you gently guide it (the great thing about toys designed specifically for anal play is that they're often tapered, making them easier to insert than, say, a penis). You'll want to stop again once you feel the resistance of the sphincter muscle just inside the rectum. Let him take a few deep breaths and as he relaxes into it, gently glide the toy in.

AT YOUR FINGERTIPS

Butt plug or anal beads

Lube

Most butt toys are designed so that, once inserted, they can be left in place (look Ma, no hands!) so that you can go about doing other things, like laundry. Kidding. Here are some things you can both do:

• Insert a butt plug in his bum while you give him a hand job or while you perform oral sex on him. Every so often, gently slide the butt plug in and out (but not all the way out) as you play with his penis.

• He wears a butt plug during intercourse and you reach behind him and use the plug to penetrate him while he is penetrating you.

• Conversely, you can experience double penetration by wearing a butt plug during intercourse.

• He can insert his fingers into your vagina and stimulate your clitoris while you're sporting a butt plug.

With you both nicely turned on and warmed up, you may well decide that tonight is the night you want to go all the way and try anal sex. Choosing the right position is the key to making your first adventure in anal sex fun and comfortable. For example, if you lie side by side, as if you were spooning, you can enter her from behind. This is a nice, relaxed position that allows you to hold her and sense if she is tensing up. If you're more confident, doggie-style (that is, her on all fours and you on your knees entering her from behind) is obviously perfectly designed for anal sex. Or try the missionary position and have her raise her pelvis by pulling her knees up toward her chest so that you have better rear-entry access. It's more difficult to change positions during anal sex than during more traditional intercourse, so experiment with different positions before you get started to see what feels best for both of you.

Once you've decided on a position and you both feel ready, squeeze a generous amount of water- or silicone-based lube or oil (though, if you're using a condom, oil will destroy the latex) onto your penis. Keep the lube handy because you'll want to add more as you go (a pump bottle is great for this). Trickle a few drops onto her bottom. There's really no such thing as too much lube when it comes to anal sex.

Quick Tip:
How Not To

Porn usually depicts anal sex as being as smooth and easy as vaginal penetration. But the fact is that (a) these women are pros who are paid to make it look easy, and (b) unless it's an anal "how-to" video, the warm-up footage is likely lying on the editing room floor.

Hold on to the base of your erect penis to give yourself plenty of control and start by circling the head around her anus to stimulate all the wonderful nerve endings located there. This will encourage her anal and sphincter muscles to relax. Press the head of your penis gently, and I mean gently, against the opening. Don't push. The moment she feels you pushing, her automatic reaction will likely be to push you out. As she breathes and relaxes, imagine her drawing you in. Remember the feeling from your experiments with fingers? Help her relax by caressing her buttocks with your hands and running your hands down her back if you're doing it doggie-style. If you're doing it missionary-style, look into her eyes, kiss her and let her know how much you love her.

Once the tip of your penis is inside her anus, you'll feel the resistance of her sphincter muscle. Again, press eeever so gently and wait for her to relax and pull you in. As her sphincter muscle starts to relax, don't mistake this for the green light to start thrusting. Hold still and let her get used to the feeling. Get her to take several deep breaths and relax her entire pelvis. She should imagine drawing you in as you gently, and again I mean gently, push your way through this muscle. When you're past the sphincter and into the rectum, that feeling of resistance will ease up. It's important that she keep breathing all the way through this. The more tense she is, the more potentially uncomfortable she will be.

Once you're all the way in, it's best to let her control the speed and depth of your thrusts until she completely relaxes and gets into it. Or not. Nothing says that once she lets you in, she has to let you stay. Again, let her control things. If she is uncomfortable or in pain, stop and perhaps try again later, or next time, or never, if that's what she decides. If she's enjoying herself, you can start to vary your thrusts. Follow a slow, deep thrust with a few quicker, shallower thrusts. Try not to pull out past the sphincter muscle. A sudden exit can be just as uncomfy as a sudden entrance and may cause her to tense up, making reentry painful or difficult. If you can reach her lady bits while deep inside her, stimulating her clitoris with your fingers will also help her

---

Quick Tip: That Depends

It's a myth that regular anal sex will sentence you to a lifetime in Depends. The anal and sphincter muscles are very strong—that's why they're so good at holding stuff inside there until you let it leave. If anal play is something you want to engage in often and you are concerned about muscle tone, you can strengthen your pelvic muscles, which support the area between the anus and the genitals and include the pubococcygeus or PC muscles. Exercise them by squeezing and releasing the entire area several times a day. Squeeze, release, squeeze, release, squeeze . . .

---

to become more aroused and loosen up. As you become more excited and closer to orgasm, the temptation to thrust deeper and faster will be hard to resist. This is less of an issue during vaginal sex, but during anal sex it becomes important to always be conscious of how she is doing, to note whether she's tensing up or getting more turned on. If she's tensing up, you need to slow down. If she seems relaxed and into it, continue. If you can't tell, ask her how she's doing. Because of the snug fit, you're more likely than she to orgasm during anal penetration. If she wants to orgasm with you inside of her, she can use her fingers or a vibrator on her clitoris.

Once you come, or you both decide you've had enough, again, exit politely. If you have climaxed, you might want to wait until you are no longer erect before pulling out. If you don't come and are still erect or semi-erect, allow her sphincter muscle to relax and let you out (remember, that's

what it's designed to do, after all). If you both came, bask in the glow and intensity of an incredibly intimate experience. If you came and she didn't, ask her if she'd like to and either help her get there or kiss and caress her while she finishes up. If neither of you had an orgasm and you decide to continue on to other sexual activities, especially vaginal penetration or fellatio, give your willy a wash to avoid the risk of transferring bacteria from the rectum area to her vagina or mouth. If you used a condom during anal sex, put on a fresh one before engaging in vaginal sex.

Of course, she doesn't always have to be the catcher. You might decide to try reversing positions. Strap-on anal sex—also known as "bend over, boyfriend" sex or "pegging" (and no, it has nothing to do with cribbage)—is not for everyone, but some couples find it intriguing. She may be turned on by the idea of switching traditional sex roles and being the one to wield the mighty sword. He may be curious about how it would feel to be "done" by her. The fact that this is taboo, fairly uncharted territory might be a turn-on for both of you.

If this is something you or your guy decide you'd like to explore, "I'd like to do you/I'd like you to do me with a strap-on, honey" probably isn't the best way to open up the dialogue. So, how do you find out if your partner is interested? Choose a time when you're both relaxed and feeling open to each other. In other words, it's probably not a good idea to suggest trying strap-on sex when you're running around getting ready to host a dinner, for example. You can mention that you've been reading about strap-ons recently and are curious about them. Or rent a porn movie that features strap-on play and see how it makes you both feel.

If you're both keen to explore, look at sex-toy catalogues together and decide on a harness and dildo combination you both think you might like. Because guys are often obsessed with their own size, they tend to head straight for the super-size dildo. A word of advice: Start small. Remind him where it is going. When you use it, follow the same instructions I gave him for butt sex with you: Take things slow, start with plenty of warm-up, use lots of lube and let him control your thrusting, drawing you in rather than you pushing your way in. Remember,

he's got a lot more experience brandishing a penis than you do. Which reminds me. There is one very important difference between his penis and yours: A strap-on dildo can't give its owner biofeedback like a real penis can, so be extra careful.

If you're serious about exploring the world of strap-on sex, there are entire books and videos devoted to the subject that offer advice beyond the limited information I have space for here. Go online or head to a reputable sex shop for some suggestions that can get you started.

- -

Quick Tip:
Play Fair

Ultimately, you can't force your partner to do something they don't want to do. The more you pressure them, the less likely you're going to convince them. And no, "If you really loved me, you'd try it" is not a fair tactic. Obviously, any sexual act is more fun and enjoyable if you're both into it. If you decide you're not into bum play, that doesn't necessarily make you uptight or closed-minded. Just because it seems like everyone else is doing it doesn't mean they are and it doesn't mean you have to do it too. There are lots of ways to enjoy a steamy, connected and even adventurous sex life without anal play. It's more important that you get the most from the sex you have, rather than expecting certain sexual acts to automatically improve your sex life. You may try anal sex and find it doesn't live up to your expectations, and that's okay.

- -

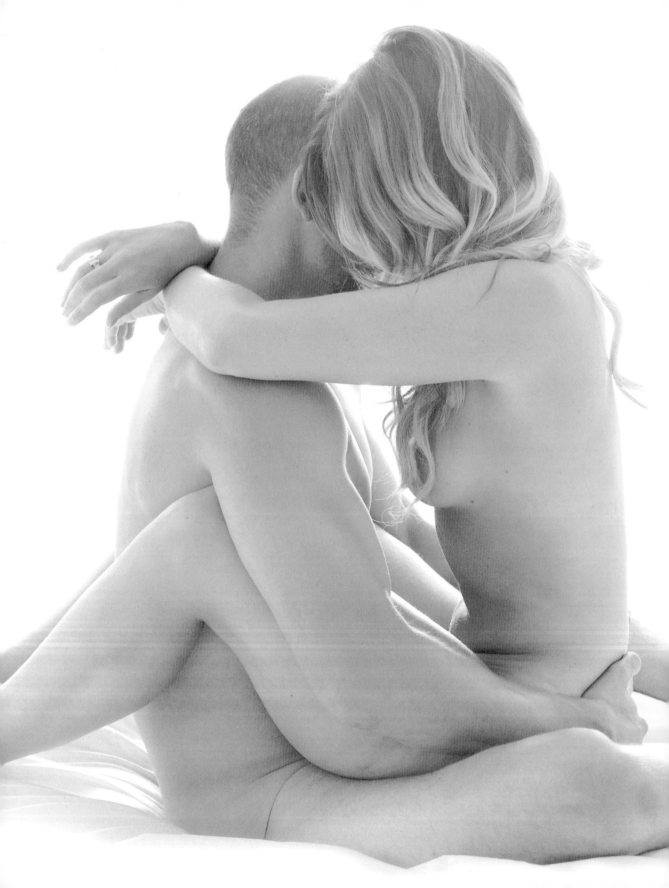

Chapter Twelve
TANTRIC

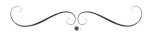

Given that for North Americans, tantric sex tends to conjure up images of Sting having seven-hour orgasms, including the topic in a sex advice book for time-strapped couples may seem contradictory. Ye of little faith. You can experiment with elements of tantric sex without learning to have sex in downward dog position while staring into each other's third eye. Aspects of tantric sex can easily be incorporated into your regular sex life. If you're simply looking to give your sex life a nifty spiritual kick in the butt, this may be all you need. If, however, after dipping your toe in the mystical waters, you discover that you are inspired to pursue this practice more seriously as a couple, go for it. There are plenty of courses, books and resources that can help you along your spiritual path.

Even if you're just dabbling, you should have at least a basic grasp of what you're dabbling in. Simply and very roughly translated, the word "Tantra" means expansion. Born in India more than six thousand years ago, Tantra was basically a reaction to Hindu and Buddhist beliefs that sex was an obstacle to enlightenment that should be avoided. Instead, tantric practitioners saw really hot sex as a route to enlightenment and transcendence. The point of tantric sex is not intercourse or even orgasm. In fact, there are no first, second or third bases in tantric sex, no beginning, middle or end. Most of the exercises related to tantric sex involve slowing things down, shifting focus away from the physicality of your body and orgasm and toward the flow of sexual energy through your body.

If you've ever practised yoga or tai chi, you may be familiar with the notion of ch'i. In the ancient East Asian belief system of Taoism, ch'i basically runs the show. It is the life force that courses through everything, including the human body. Keeping ch'i flowing freely throughout your body is believed to do many things: restore balance, cure illness and open up your heart and spirit. If you think of sexual energy in terms of ch'i, keeping it flowing throughout your body can have the same effects on your sex life. There are mental and physical exercises designed to tap into your sexual

energy and move it throughout your body rather than keeping it all crammed in your genital area. Practising these exercises on a regular basis can bring your sexual experiences together to new heights, deepening and expanding your sexual connection.

TIME to PLAY

Five Minutes or Less
Don't Stop Staring at Me

When you wake up together, take a few moments to really look at each other before you start your day. Spend a minute or so drinking in your partner's face and breathing quietly together. After a minute of soft, slow breathing, practise something known in tantric circles as a "charging breath." Together, breathe in and out rapidly ten times and follow this with one slow, deep breath. Repeat this pattern ten times together. This will awaken your energies and "charge" you for the day.

Squeeze Me

One of the beliefs associated with tantric sex is that ejaculation depletes your energy. Tantric practitioners believe that exercising the pubococcygeus muscles (also known as the PC or "love" muscles) can help delay ejaculation and intensify your orgasms. Same goes for women (well, not the delaying ejaculation part but the intensifying part). It can also help keep things nice and snug down there, a concern for a lot of women, especially after childbirth. The easiest way to locate your PC muscles is to stop mid-pee. Congratulations, you just did your first rep. Squeeze . . . and . . . release . . . squeeze . . . release. Do this twenty to thirty times a day, whenever you have some time to kill, like when standing in line at the grocery store, waiting for the bus . . .

The Tantric Quickie

I know, that seems like the ultimate oxymoron given that most of what we hear about tantric sex is about prolonging pleasure and lasting forever. But one of the practices tantric teachers encourage is to make love first thing in the morning without wasting any time on silly things like foreplay. Tomorrow morning, spend a minute or so stimulating each other just enough to make penetration possible. Have intercourse, facing each other, eyes open, for a few minutes. Neither of you may experience orgasm but that's not the point (in fact, he should try not to ejaculate). The point is to connect physically and spiritually. This will heighten your sexual energy, give you practice at being "ready" any time (especially important for women), and train him to last longer and feel his sexual energy without expending it. It'll also leave you both horny, so there will be lots of yummy leftover sexual tension hanging around between you.

One Hour or Less
Don't Hold Your Breath

It's as simple as breathing. No, really. One of the simplest ways to intensify sex is to improve your breathing. If you've ever taken yoga, you know how often the instructor reminds you to breathe. Tonight, pay attention to your breathing while you're having sex. You'll notice that, as you become more sexually excited, your breath gets quick and shallow. As you near orgasm, you may even hold your breath completely for several moments at a time. If you notice this happening, pause and focus on changing your breathing. Breathe in deeply through your nose and feel the air move down to your chest and right into your pelvic area and genitals. Visualize the sexual energy flowing through your body as you do this. You may be surprised at how much this allows you to open up and let go during sex.

If you find this exercise helpful, you may want to practise breathing in sync. You can sit facing each other on the bed to do this, naked or not. Start with soft, deep breaths while looking into each other's eyes. This may make you self-conscious or want to laugh, but try to stay with it. Start breathing at the same pace, slowly in through your nose and out your mouth.

Maintain eye contact. Keep practising until you can maintain harmonized breathing for five minutes. It may feel like five hours at first but again, try and stay with it: Start with a shorter period and increase the time as you get more comfortable. Feel your breath in sync and the sexual energy flowing between you.

Practise this exercise as you kiss as well, but rather than breathing in sync, breathe in through your nose and release your breath into your partner's mouth. On the receiving end, relax and imagine the breath moving down deep into your body as you breathe in, and then release your breath back into your partner's mouth. Breathe back and forth like this until you feel the sexual energy moving between your mouths, or you feel like you're going to pass out. Whichever comes first.

Tune In and Turn On

Spiritual sex is about being present and aware of your senses. Besides focusing on your breath, other simple things can increase your spiritual presence and intensify the sexual energy between you as a couple. The next time you have sex:

Open Your Eyes

You may be surprised to realize how often you keep your eyes closed during sex. Closing your eyes can certainly help you focus and shut out distraction. But something as simple as opening your eyes during intercourse can be incredibly powerful. (Imagine staring warmly and deeply into each other's souls as opposed to freaky "what are you looking at?" staring.) Even while kissing, opening your eyes and looking at each other can create an even stronger sense of connection and intensity.

Listen

The sound of sex can be incredibly arousing. Enthusiastic moaning, groaning, even letting loose with a heartfelt "yeah, baby" or some slightly more expressive phrases can be a total turn-on. But sometimes it can feel like a bit of a performance. Try turning off the porno soundtrack once in a while and let your breath be the soundtrack. Listen to the sharp intake of her breath as you enter her. Tune in to the sounds of your bodies slapping together or his wet tongue lapping your vulva. Instead of forcing it, allow any moaning or groaning to be released naturally.

Stay Still

So much time during sex is wasted worrying about your next move—what to put where and when and how. All that moving around can be distracting and stop you from really feeling one another. Learn to be still. After you enter her, don't start thrusting immediately. Just hold yourself inside her as you both relish the feeling of your bodies being literally connected. If you are performing oral sex on him, hold him deep in your mouth and savour your warm breath and mouth on his penis. When you are going down on her, close your mouth over her clitoris and just hold it there for as long as you can. Relax and simply feel his warm breath and wet mouth on you and imagine his sexual energy flowing from his mouth through your clitoris and then throughout your entire body.

Don't Make It About Orgasm

Decide beforehand that neither of you will focus on giving each other an orgasm. Removing orgasm from the playing field altogether allows you both to be in the moment rather than focusing on whether you're getting there or not.

How Chakra-ing!

The philosophy behind acupressure, Tantra and other Eastern-based practices is that you can release energy by applying pressure to certain energy points on the body called chakras. These points include the pubic bone (the area of the pelvis just above the genitals), the lower back, the middle of the chest, the throat, the spot on the forehead between the eyes, and the top of the head. Massaging each of these areas releases sexual energy throughout the body.

You don't have to have extensive knowledge of Eastern philosophy or even know precisely where or what these energy points are in order to pay special attention to these areas as part of your regular sexual routine. While you're in the missionary position, for example, wrap your hand around the base of her head and slide it down her neck, gently but firmly squeezing your thumb and forefinger together. Imagine drawing sexual energy from her head down into her upper back and chest area. While you have his penis in one hand, run your other hand firmly down the front of his thighs, imagining the sexual energy being pulled from his groin down through his legs. Focusing your attention on these other sexual energy points while you are being intimate will help you to experience a more intense, spiritual and full-body sexual connection.

All Night

Yab-yummy Evening

Tantric sex practitioners are a clean bunch. Most tantric sexual practices start with some kind of bathing ritual. To put it simply, the belief behind this is that your partner's body is sacred and it's pretty much your duty to honour and cherish it. Turning the act of bathing each other into a fancy-schmancy event is a lovely, sensual way to do this. You'll also feel more confident

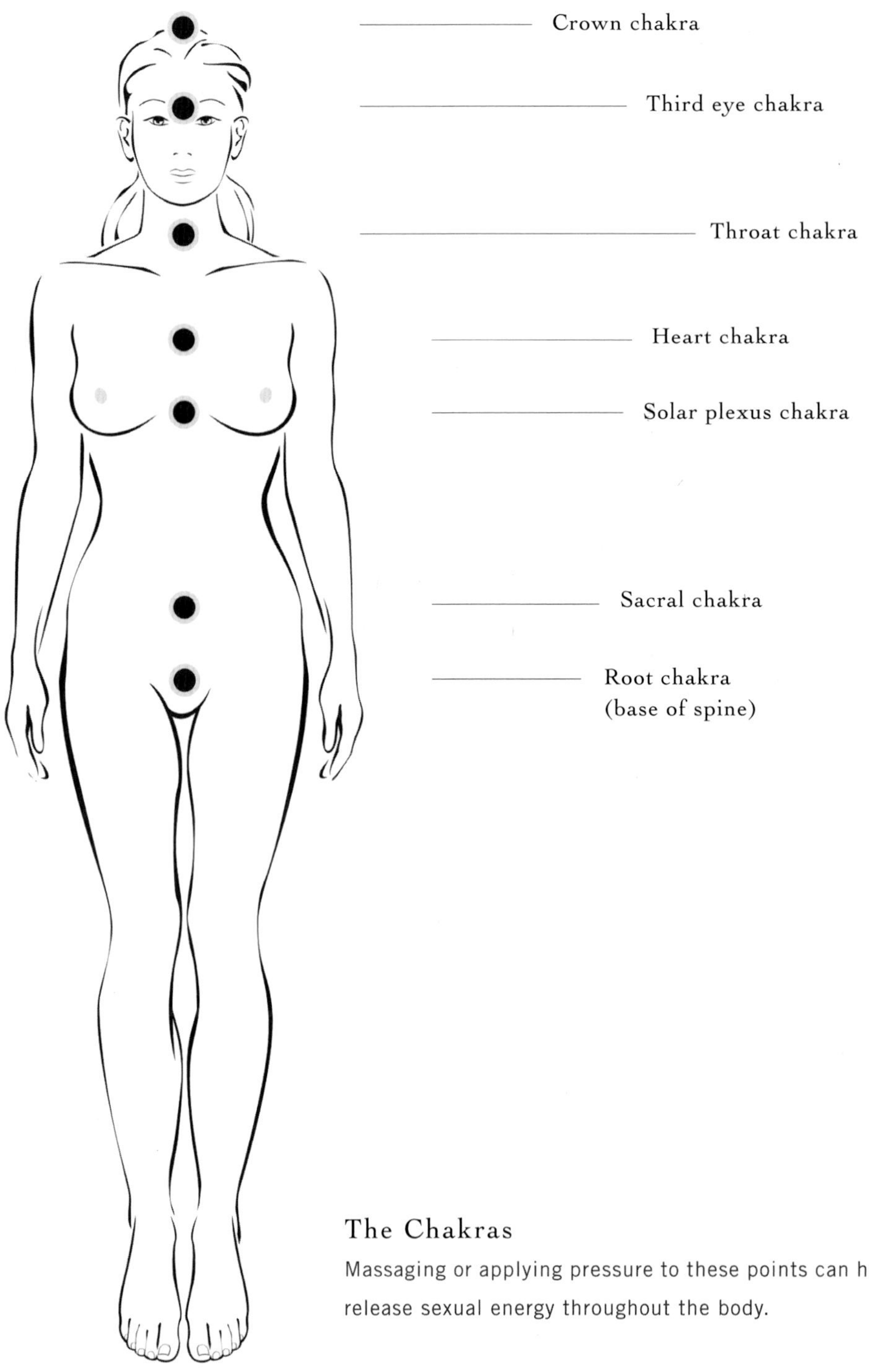

Crown chakra

Third eye chakra

Throat chakra

Heart chakra

Solar plexus chakra

Sacral chakra

Root chakra
(base of spine)

The Chakras

Massaging or applying pressure to these points can help release sexual energy throughout the body.

exploring each other's chakras when your own are clean as a whistle.

AT YOUR FINGERTIPS

Fluffy bathrobes

Candles

Soothing music

Chilled bubbly

Scented bath oil

Washcloth

Fancy soap or shower gel

Shampoo

So start your enchanted tantric evening with a cleansing bath. Don't simply turn on the taps and go watch TV while the tub fills. Spend time setting the mood together by first cleaning the bathroom and tub, getting rid of any clutter and wayward kids' bath toys, and laying out a couple of plush towels and some body lotion for when you get out. Turn up the heat so the room is nice and cozy and get into your bathrobes. As you run the bath, add some scented bath salts or oils to the water, light some candles, get some mood music happening and chill a bottle of wine or even some bubbly in an ice bucket. Slowly remove each other's bathrobes and spend some time kissing and caressing (not too much of that though, we've still got a whole bath to get through here).

Lower yourselves into the water so that you sit facing each other and then enjoy a glass of bubbly as you spend a few quiet moments simply taking in the environment and your partner. Use your favourite soap or shower gel and a fluffy washcloth, and take time washing each other from head to toe. Pay attention to how your slippery, soapy hands feel as they glide across your partner's body. Wash each other's hair. (If you don't have a bathtub, showering together can also be turned into a sensual bathing ritual. Simply take the same tender care in washing each other. The most important thing is that you are lavishing attention on each other.)

When you are finished bathing and sufficiently pruney, step out of the bath and tenderly dry each other with the towels you've put out, then slather each other with body lotion, massaging each area as you rub the cream into your partner's skin. Once you are both well moisturized and cozy back in your bathrobes, grab the rest of the champagne and head to your bed, where you can decide what to do with your ritually cleansed, relaxed and spiritually connected bodies. You may want to simply snuggle together and fall asleep in each other's arms, feed each other in bed (sharing food is another important tantric ritual), indulge your partner in a full-body massage or make sweet love to each other.

Quick Tip:
Scentsual

Certain scents are believed to enhance your libido. During your tantric sessions, burn musk, sandalwood or jasmine incense.

If you decide on the latter, put a tantric twist on your lovemaking tonight with the yab-yum position, which allows you to incorporate many of the practices I've described in this section. He sits cross-legged on the bed or floor. She sits in his lap, facing him with her legs wrapped around his bum and the bottoms of her feet pressed together behind him (if her butt in your lap is uncomfy for either of you, slip a pillow under her bottom). In this position, your eyes and hearts are facing, and you can maintain eye contact, kiss and hug as you make love. The other tantric benefit of this position for him is that it allows for deep penetration, so he should have no trouble maintaining arousal, but it prevents him from being able to thrust too vigorously, helping to delay ejaculation.

But he's not the only one who can reap the tantric benefits of this position. There are a few things you can do to help intensify the connection. Rather than thrusting your pelvis toward him, rock it back and forth (pull your pelvis up toward your ribs and then push your bum down) while he is deep inside. Rock quickly and then slowly. Stay still and look directly into his eyes, concentrating on the feeling of him inside you and focusing on the energy flowing between you.

As I've mentioned, orgasm isn't the focus in tantric sex, but if she comes, that's okay (just don't force it). Sorry mister, but in tantric sex, the woman gets to come as much as she wants because her "life force," unlike yours, isn't spent when she does. See, in tantric sex, the ultimate goal is for the man to orgasm without ejaculation. The thinking behind this is that your unejaculated semen is reabsorbed into your body, thereby retaining your sexual energy and vitality instead of spilling it all over her stomach.

With a lot of training and practice, you can learn ejaculatory control and, like an expert surfer, you can learn to ride the crest of your orgasm wave without tipping over. Maybe even more than once, and you won't even need a surfboard, just a lot of breathing, patience and a strong set of PC muscles. When you feel your arousal getting stronger during sex, stop whatever you're doing (if you're inside her, stop thrusting and just rest). Relax and focus on your breathing and your partner until your arousal subsides enough to continue. Visualize redirecting the sexual energy from your penis up and throughout your entire body. Imagine a sexy current circling from your head down to your crotch, through her genitals, up to her head and vice versa.

Go back to thrusting and, when your arousal crests again, stop, relax, visualize, focus on your breath and on her. If you wait too long and start to feel that orgasmic wave about to come over you, pump your PC muscles to stop yourself from going over the brink. You can also pull your boys down and away from your body—known in tantric circles as the "testes tug"—or squeeze your penis just below the head to help stop impending orgasm. Keep practising, using all of these techniques every time you have sex or even when you masturbate and, in time, you just might be able to come like a girl—that is, without ejaculating.

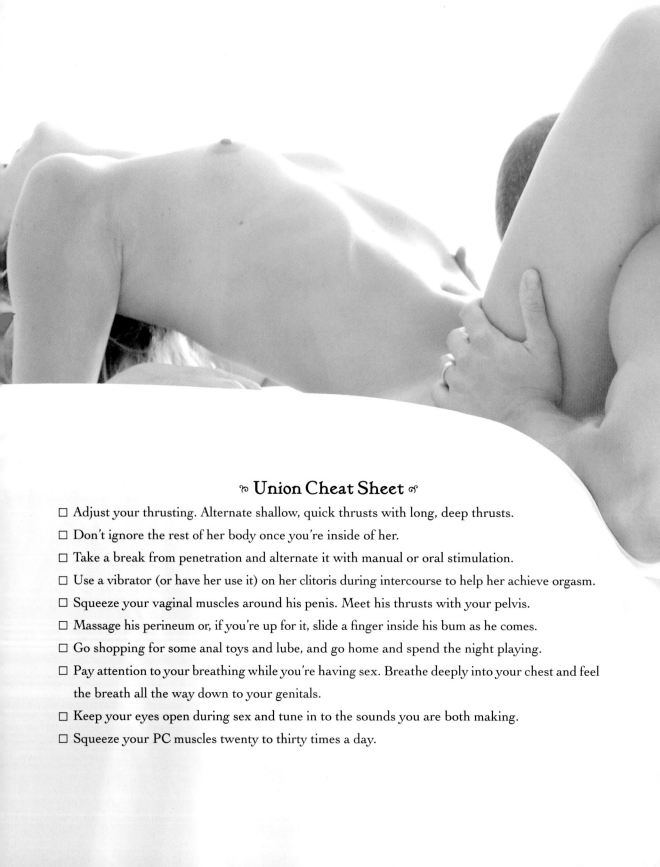

❧ Union Cheat Sheet ❧

☐ Adjust your thrusting. Alternate shallow, quick thrusts with long, deep thrusts.

☐ Don't ignore the rest of her body once you're inside of her.

☐ Take a break from penetration and alternate it with manual or oral stimulation.

☐ Use a vibrator (or have her use it) on her clitoris during intercourse to help her achieve orgasm.

☐ Squeeze your vaginal muscles around his penis. Meet his thrusts with your pelvis.

☐ Massage his perineum or, if you're up for it, slide a finger inside his bum as he comes.

☐ Go shopping for some anal toys and lube, and go home and spend the night playing.

☐ Pay attention to your breathing while you're having sex. Breathe deeply into your chest and feel the breath all the way down to your genitals.

☐ Keep your eyes open during sex and tune in to the sounds you are both making.

☐ Squeeze your PC muscles twenty to thirty times a day.

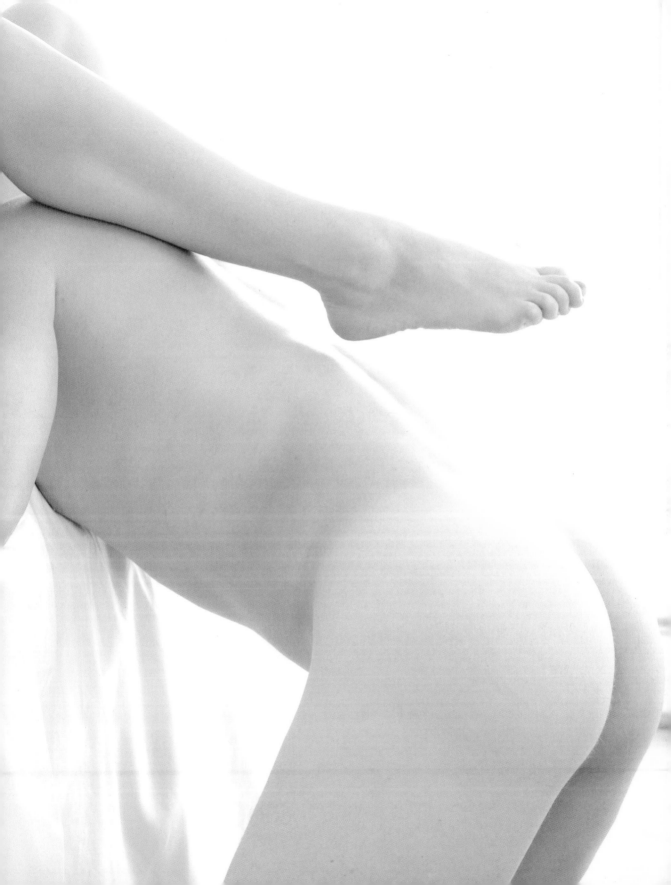

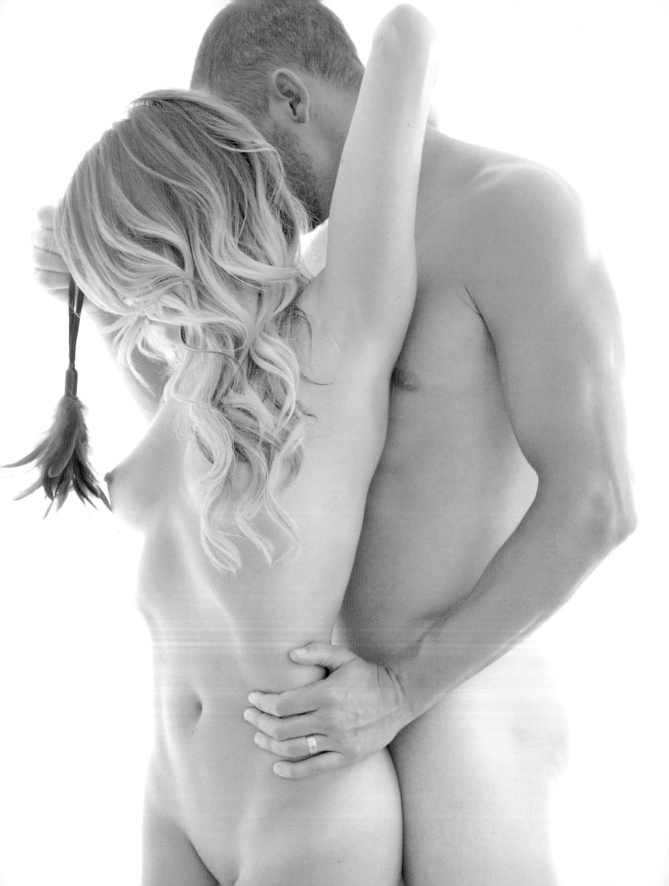

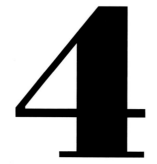

SPICE

I think you're ready to take things up a notch. Adding a little novelty to your sex life will keep things fresh, inventive and challenging, keeping the two of you interested, intrigued and, thus, inspired. Don't worry, I'm not going to suggest you turn your basement into a dungeon or run out and buy yourself a full set of bullwhips. I'm just talking about some more adventurous sex play to shake things up. Admittedly, if you've seen media images of people in leather hoods and head-to-toe latex brandishing whips and chains, role-play and bondage might strike you as weird or even scary, but don't let that intimidate you. You can explore the world of fantasy and kink without either of you wearing a collar and leash or licking anyone's boots. Besides, "weird" is a relative term. What's so weird about having consensual, connected, exciting, adventurous sex in the privacy of your own home where you aren't harming anyone? Scary? I don't doubt it. It's much safer and less frightening to stay in your predictable sexual rut. But if you wanted to do that, you wouldn't be reading this, would you?

Here I suggest some fun, simple ways to incorporate fantasy into your lives and I guide you through more elaborate fantasy material like role-playing and threesomes. On the kinky side of things, I teach you how you can add just a dash of spice to make your regular sex life a little less vanilla. And, for when you're feeling more adventurous, I show you the ropes, quite literally, as I guide you through a basic bondage session. You'll learn how to give your sweetheart a good spanking and, finally, how to get bossy with some basic dominance/submission training.

Time Challenge

If you have ten seconds . . .
Give her bum a quick swat as you pass her on the stairs. Follow this with a passionate kiss on the lips.

If you have one minute . . .
Let yourself fantasize about anything or anyone you want. No one needs to know.

If you have ten minutes . . .
Tell your partner about one type of extreme sexual play you're curious about and ask them what they think about it.

If you have half an hour . . .
Put your hair up in a bun, wear a pair of glasses and play "teacher" as you instruct him on how to pleasure you orally.

If you have an hour . . .
If you're usually the bossy one in your relationship, tell your partner you'll do anything they tell you to for the whole hour.

If you have all night . . .
Tie his wrists and ankles to a chair and "torture" him as you slowly strip naked and then tease his entire body with your mouth and hands.

START WITH THE BASICS

Be up front.

When delving into uncharted sexual territory, it's essential to talk first.
When doing so, stay open, don't be pushy and don't pass judgment.

Establish and respect boundaries.

No matter how badly you would like to try something, your partner may not
wish to go there. Honour this feeling and do not pressure them.

Be extra sensitive.

Delving into intensely physical and potentially psychological sexual play requires
lots of trust and communication. You both need to feel safe and
understood for it to go well.

Don't be too rigid.

It may be that your partner's into experimenting but just not in the way
you're suggesting, at least for starters. The experiment is more likely to go well
if you start with something that you both agree upon.

Consider trying one bite.

Think back to when you were a kid and didn't want to try a new food.
Your mom told you to at least eat a bite before you decided for sure you didn't like
it. You may surprise yourself. Maybe getting tied up and giving up control
while your partner devotes all their attention and energy to your pleasure
might not be such a bad thing after all.

Pay attention.

Be aware of your partner's body language and any feedback that indicates they are
uncomfortable, in real pain or just not into it. If they want you to stop, stop.

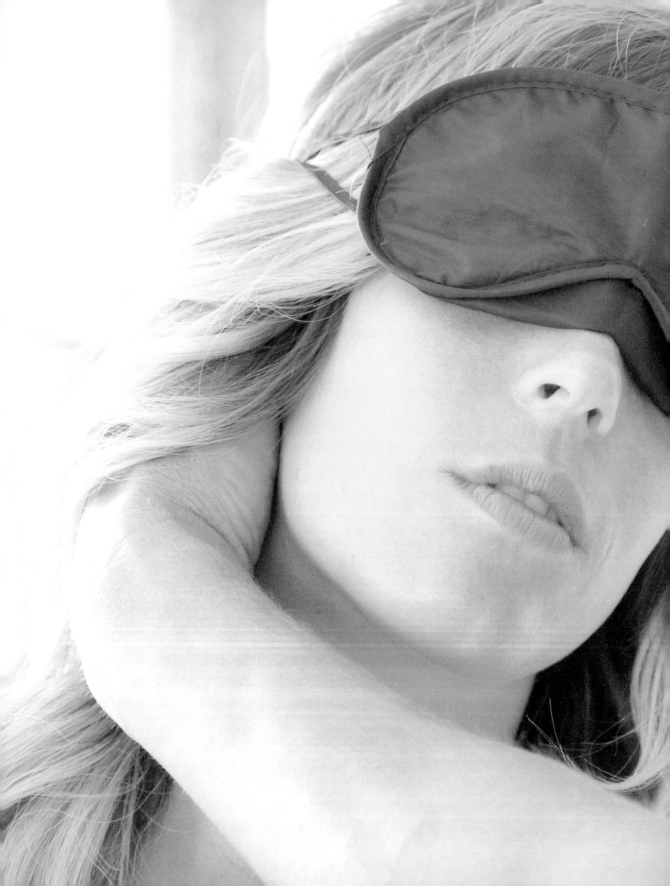

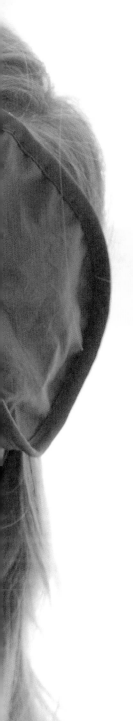

Chapter Thirteen
FANTASY

You're masturbating to an image in your head of him entering you from behind. You find yourself drifting off at work and remembering the last time she went down on you. You think about being tied to the bed and having to totally give up control while he strokes, licks and teases every part of your body. You imagine her dressed up as a schoolgirl who needs to be disciplined.

From brief sexual thoughts—just thinking about his warm tongue on your nipple or her hot breath against the head of your penis—to more extreme scenarios—her in full dominatrix gear towering over you with a whip—fantasy is a great way to flick on your brain's sex switch.

Fantasy is all about adventure and pretending, much like when you were a kid, but R-rated. It can provide a wonderful break from reality, fuel your sexual imagination, give you permission to be someone or something other than who you are, and let you experience things you may never have the chance to experience—or may not even want to experience—in real life.

Fantasies can be scary or uncomfortable because they may not be politically correct or may go against your usual nature. You know violence against women is wrong but you fantasize about being tied up and taken by force. You're in a happy, monogamous relationship but get turned on by the idea of sex with someone else. You consider yourself a straight woman but fantasize about performing cunnilingus. As a result, it can be tempting to quell your fantasies, perhaps because you are ashamed or embarrassed by them. Sadly, in doing so you also quell your sexual imagination and your sense of sexual adventure, and cheat yourself out of one of the best ways to explore new sexual horizons. So don't let fantasy scare you.

The thing to remember is that you are in control. You get to write the script. Let me show you: Okay, imagine meeting George Clooney. In your head, he's completely charmed by you and invites you to stay with him at his villa in Italy for a week,

after which he's so smitten with you that he doesn't want you to leave. Of course, if you met George Clooney in real life, he'd probably flash you that fantastic grin as he politely tried to back away from the crazy lady telling him how absolutely gorgeous and handsome and charming and amazing she thinks he is. Sigh.

Ahem, anyway.

Because fantasies are so private in nature, revealing them to a partner can make you feel extremely vulnerable. For this reason, sharing fantasies requires tremendous trust. That's also why it's hot. Letting your partner in on your dirty little secrets is extremely intimate and daring. And, as with most things in life, the bigger the risk, the greater the reward.

I'm not saying you need to give it all away. There may be fantasies you never share with your partner, something private that helps get you off while masturbating, for example, and that's fine. But in other cases, verbalizing a few of your fantasies is a quick and easy way to venture into unexplored sexual territory. Your fantasy life together can be as simple or as complex as you both want to make it. While I touch on several common fantasies in this section, by nature fantasy is only limited by your imagination. Use these ideas as inspiration, but feel free to let your sexual imagination run wild.

TIME to PLAY

Five Minutes or Less

Flash Fantasy

Write down one fantasy each and swap. (If you need inspiration, see the list of top male and female fantasies in "Playbook K: Fantasy Material" on pages 218–20.) Read each other's fantasies in private so you have time to sit with your reaction and then jot down your response. Give one of three responses: "Sorry, honey, not my thing," "Intrigued, but makes me shy or nervous," or "Oh, yeah, that's hot." Swap responses. It's not important whether you ever act on these fantasies; the point of this exercise is to get you both more comfortable sharing.

Hotter Than the Licence Plate Game

Revealing that you have a secret desire to be tied up and taken against your will might not be appropriate dinner conversation, especially if the kids are around. Long (kid-free) car rides are a good opportunity to share, as are walks in the park, on the beach, in the country—any neutral, relaxed, private environment where you're both feeling safe and connected.

On your next car trip alone together, play a fantasy game. One of you comes up with a person, a place, an object and an action, and the other person has to create a saucy story using all the suggestions. If you have trouble coming up with a fantasy,

replay a past sexual encounter between the two of you and go into detail about what you liked about it. By revealing what stood out for you in the encounter you also reveal some of the things you fantasize about. Take it one step further and elaborate on the scene, adding some details from your own private fantasy stash. If you're describing a particularly memorable oral sex session, for example, and you've always fantasized about having your hands tied while he pleasures you orally, toss it in there. Or tell her about a sexy dream you had about her and describe in detail what she was doing to you. Hot and instructional.

Dress Up

Search your closet and put together your best naughty schoolgirl outfit, take a picture of yourself and text it to him. Replace naughty schoolgirl with naughty housewife (apron, heels, nothing else), naughty nurse (pick up a tight uniform at a second-hand shop) or just plain naughty (stockings, garter, stilettos).

One Hour or Less

Sexy Story Time

A fantastic way to explore fantasy is through erotic stories. The erotica market has exploded in recent years, and you can find collections of stories with themes ranging from vampire-inspired erotica to lesbian cowgirl erotica. This range allows you to experience sex vicariously through various sexual orientations and sexual preferences. You may never delve into the world of BDSM (short for bondage and discipline, dominance and submission, and sadism and masochism, as explained more fully in the "Kink" chapter) beyond tying him to the bed with a silk scarf, but you can experience and be aroused by that world through erotica. And, unlike onscreen porn, erotica lets you create the visuals in your own mind. It allows you to expand your sexual imagination and can inspire you to incorporate new things into your sex life. It's a great way to discover your partner's turn-ons (and turn-offs) as well as some of your own. Plus, reading sexy stories to each other will no doubt get you both pretty randy.

Quick Tip:
Fair Share

Even if your partner's fantasy freaks you out a little, try to open your heart and your mind. Remember, fantasies are about imagination and imaginations can be wild. They don't necessarily have anything to do with reality. And there is no rule that telling each other your fantasies means you have to act on them. In fact, simply describing them in excruciating detail to one another can be hot in its own right. And this sharing may be all the sparkle your sex life needs for now.

Many larger Canadian cities now have at least one cool sex shop where you will find a good selection of erotica and a knowledgeable staff who can help you pick a few titles to get you started, depending on your interests. Even large mainstream bookstores now have erotica sections, though the staff will be less knowledgeable about the quality, so you may want to search their selection online. There are also several online sites that publish erotic stories you can download. Search "erotica for couples." Once you've found some material you like, tell her that tonight after you tuck in the kids and read them a bedtime story, you've got a special bedtime story for her. When you are snuggled in bed together, read your sexy story aloud.

Shopping for Pleasure

Beyond erotica, browsing through a sex shop together provides a great opportunity to explore the world of fantasy and to discover what piques each other's curiosity, from toys to outfits to accessories and even pornography. Leave the judgment at home, go in with an open mind and have fun with it (if you've ever wondered what your fella would look like in a French maid outfit, here's your chance). Seek out a sex shop with an experienced staff that will make you feel comfortable and at ease (see the "Toys" appendix for more info on sex shops). If you want to explore porn, for example, but have no idea what to look for, they can guide you through the maze of titles, genres, even directors to help you find something you both might like. Even if you leave the store with nothing, the experience will help you to open up and talk about the things you're intrigued by when it comes to fantasy.

Arousing Browsing

Spend time surfing the Internet together. Start by simply typing "sex fantasies" into your favourite search engine and see what you find. There are tons of sites with stories, images and ideas for couples, so use the opportunity to open up to each other about your fantasies. If you see something that sparks your sexual interest, say so. Keep an open mind and resist judgment. Be warned, any time you type "sex" into an Internet search engine, you're bound to stumble across a few sites that make you uncomfortable. It's okay, you don't have to visit them. Talk about what you're seeing and how it makes you feel. If something excites the two of you — be it a story or certain images — act on your feelings. Mutually masturbate, go down on him while he reads what's on the screen, or go down on her while she describes what's exciting her.

All Night

Given more time, there are a number of ways you could explore fantasy, so I've provided three different all-night scenarios for you to try.

Porn to Be Wild

Spend an evening watching porn together. I know, a lot of porn is cheesy and embarrassing and not particularly realistic, but it can play a role in your sex life. On a basic level, watching other people have sex can be a real turn-on, and watching it as a couple may simply get you both horny. It can also teach you a lot about each other's sexual curiosities, likes, dislikes and boundaries.

Most of us carry around a lot of cultural baggage about porn. She may have grown up thinking it's degrading to women and still feel that way. He may feel guilty about liking porn or feel uncomfortable about sharing what has always been a private indulgence. So you might feel awkward or shy about watching it together. Here's how to make the experience a positive one for you both:

Find Porn You Both Like

There is an increasing market for porn aimed specifically at couples that features genuine female pleasure and orgasms as well as better production values and storylines.

She may prefer this. Or she may want wall-to-wall hardcore action. Like I said, watching porn can teach you a thing or two about each other's turn-ons.

Let Her Pick

This allows her to feel like this is something new you are sharing together rather than you trying to get her on board with the kind of material that's been getting you off since you were eighteen.

Ensure You Have Privacy

Lock the door if the kids are home, or send them to grandma's. Close the curtains, dim the lights, make some popcorn. . . .

Fool Around First

You may want to make out a bit before you turn on the movie to put you in a more sexually open frame of mind. At the very least, get naked and snuggle up.

Use It as an Opportunity to Talk About Sex

Sometimes it's easier to point at something on the screen and say, "Oooh, I like how he's doing that to her," than to explain exactly how you like to be pleasured.

Let It Inspire You

No, really. Seeing something onscreen that the two of you have never tried provides an opportunity to gauge how you both feel about trying it. Then, if you're both game, give it a whirl.

Be Conscious of Each Other's Reactions

Watching a bunch of people who are paid to look good naked and have sex on camera can be a little intimidating. If she gets uncomfortable or starts feeling insecure, reassure her that the turn-on is not about wanting to have sex with the woman onscreen but the fact that you are sharing the experience with each other and then get to have real-life sex together.

Don't Take It Too Seriously

Porn can be hilariously fake and over-the-top ridiculous sometimes. You're allowed to laugh. This will help ease any tension and give you another opportunity to talk about what's going on, even if just to make fun of it together.

The Remote Control Is Your Friend

Just like when you watch alone and skip through the parts you don't like, skip through bits that bug one or both of you or that simply don't turn you on.

Making a Scene

You haven't acted since your high-school play, but tonight you and your sweetie want to dust off your acting skills and try out some role-play. Before you don your schoolgirl uniform and he his headmaster outfit, you need to think about a few things. While exciting, role-play can make you feel very vulnerable. That's part of what makes it hot, but it's also what scares most of us off. It's crucial that you both feel supported and encouraged, not judged. And that you know the only laughing will be with you, not at you. I mean it.

Whenever you're venturing into new territory, respect is the key. Role-playing can surprise you sometimes by stirring up unexpected emotions and reactions once you're in character. Take things slow, check in with each other along the way to make sure you're both okay, and stop whenever either of you feels uncomfortable. Continue this respect once play is over. It's a good idea to take some time to talk about how things went, what you liked, what was weird, what you would change if you were to do it again. Finally, don't forget to clean up your toys. It might be a little embarrassing if Mom drops by and wonders why there's a cheerleader outfit lying on your bed when it's nowhere near Halloween.

All right, with that out of the way, on with the show!

A simple way to role-play is to swap roles. If he usually takes the lead, force yourself to initiate. It may feel awkward or out of character, but the whole point of role-playing is to leave your comfort zone. I know, dressing up and playing a character is bound to make a lot of people feel ridiculous. The more in character you are, the easier it will be to make the leap, get out of your own head and play the role. Costumes are great for this. A dominatrix doesn't don a latex catsuit, high boots and a whip just for visual effect (though that's definitely an added bonus); the outfit helps her feel powerful and enact her role. You don't necessarily need to put together an entire costume. A pair of glasses and a pencil skirt might be enough to make you feel like the "hot librarian." A blonde wig if you're a brunette or a pair of stilettos when you usually wear sneakers can be enough to make you alter the way you act. If he's usually a button-down shirt kind of guy, tossing on a cowboy belt and holster with nothing else may be just the thing to make him feel like rustlin' you into the sack.

Introducing a Third Party

A threesome is a common fantasy for both men and women. Of course, like with a lot of fantasies, most couples never act on this one. Which is totally fine. Just painting the picture for each other can be a huge turn-on. In fact, playing out this fantasy verbally from time to time may create enough excitement for the two of you that you never need to act on it.

If, however, you're keen to realize this fantasy (and based on the letters I get on this topic from couples, plenty of you are), be sure you know what you're getting into.

The key to making a threesome work—as with most things sexual, but especially activities that take you out of your sexual comfort zone—is communication. Feelings of jealousy and insecurity may still take you by surprise, but at least if you've talked about them beforehand, you will be more psychologically prepared to deal with them. Talk to each other about the idea. What turns you on about a threesome? How do you imagine it playing out? How would you handle it if you got jealous or realized the reality wasn't living up to the fantasy?

If your relationship and sex life are not on a solid footing, trying to solve things by bringing a third party into your bed is a bit like having kids to save a marriage. Okay, I probably shouldn't be talking about kids and threesomes in the same sentence, but my point is that involving a third person in an already problematic situation is only going to further strain your relationship.

Ask yourself these questions:

• Are you sure you can handle watching another person kissing and having oral sex or intercourse with your partner?

• Are the two of you truly open, honest and secure in your emotional, sexual and physical relationship?

• Are you totally confident that it would take more than seeing your partner enjoy sex with another person (in your presence and with your approval, of course) to break your bond?

• Are you clear that this is about sex, not about having a relationship or falling in love with someone else?

> 66 The key to making a threesome work is communication. 99

If you're sure you're both ready, there are a couple logistical things to consider. Adding a third is not only an emotional but also a physical challenge. As the old saying goes, "Two's company, three's a crowd." Often, while the idea of a threesome might be exciting for all parties involved, the reality is quite different. Most of us have our hands full—quite literally—with just one lover. Chances are, with a threesome, someone is going to feel left out some of the time. You need to discuss the ground rules going in. Establish a word or phrase—"Hey, what about me?" is basic and direct—that any of you can use when feeling left out so you all press pause, assess the situation and do what needs to be done, talked about or shared before pressing play again. And finally, if there are things you think you might be uncomfortable with, speak up beforehand. If you're inviting another woman into your bed but don't want her kissing your guy on the lips, for example, set that rule beforehand.

Once you've established all the ground rules, you may find it less awkward to start the festivities by making out as a couple first and letting your third join in when they feel ready or when you decide to invite them. Beyond this, the mechanics are similar to any sexual encounter except with a few extra body parts. The most important thing to remember is that everyone should be respectful and know they can stop at any time if they feel left out, awkward, turned off or uncomfortable in any way. Afterward,

talk about how you all feel, especially you and your partner. Did everyone have a good time? If not, why not? If so, what did you like about it? If communication is the key to a successful relationship, it's even more important when that relationship suddenly has an extra body attached to it.

If you're not sure you want to make this fantasy a reality, there are ways to enjoy the idea of a threesome without physically inviting someone else into your bed:

• Watch some porn together that includes threesomes.

• Compose a mock personal ad together describing what you'd both be looking for if you were looking for a third person to join you.

• Go to a strip club together and buy her a lap dance.

Quick Tip: Finding Number Three

There's no real magic to finding a third party. The easiest way is to advertise, and plenty of avenues both on- and off-line cater specifically to this search. Many online dating and adult social networking sites have special sections for couples looking for a third. Some couples don't like the idea of inviting a stranger to join them and say friends are the way to go because there is a level of familiarity and comfort. Of course, other couples will tell you they have a rule about not having threesomes with friends because there is too much familiarity and it always gets weird. Some couples meet people in bars or through other social avenues and slowly reveal their agenda as they get to know the person in hopes they might be game for a threesome.

PLAYBOOK K
FANTASY MATERIAL

As inspiration, here are some of the most common themes for female and male fantasies:

HERS

Being Dominated

She may be all about equality outside the bedroom, but sometimes she imagines you throwing her down on the bed and ravishing her. (Yes, "ravish" just says it best. She wants to be ravished by you.) This is less about you controlling her than her giving up control and surrendering to you.

Dominating

Many women still have a hard time taking control in the bedroom. Taking total charge — forcing you to go down on her until she comes, making you beg for release, having you worship her, being in control and having your total attention and devotion — can be very freeing and exciting.

Sex with a Stranger

Good girls don't go home with strangers, right? Given this cultural expectation, it's not surprising that many women fantasize about picking up a stranger and taking him home for a steamy night of no-strings-attached sex.

Being Watched

Women are used to being looked at in our society, and not always in ways that they appreciate. So the idea of being watched in a way that she chooses can be very exciting. Being the object of your devoted gaze as she undresses or having you videotape or photograph her allows her to control her own image and project her sexuality as she wants to be perceived. The idea of others watching the two of you having sex appeals to her, in part, because she's thinking, "I know you want me, but only he gets to have me," and that kind of power can be a real turn-on.

Being Taken Against Her Will

Though this is often referred to as a rape fantasy, I prefer to think of it as being taken against her will because I honestly don't think any woman really fantasizes about being violently and brutally raped. The idea of being taken against her will differs slightly from being dominated in that instead of surrendering immediately, she puts up a fight. The friction as she resists while you tear off her clothes and overpower her can make for some wicked sexual tension. The fact that it goes against what is socially acceptable also lends it that reliably hot taboo flavour.

Sex with Another Woman

For a straight woman, thinking about being with another woman sexually lets her imagine what it must feel like for you to be with her. Cunnilingus, nipple play, penetration with fingers or a toy, these are things she only experiences as a receiver. The idea of experiencing it from your perspective pretty much rocks.

Sex with More Than One Man

What woman doesn't want to be showered with sexual attention? Having one man playing with her breasts while another plays with her clitoris, another penetrates her and another, I don't know, vacuums the house and feeds her grapes—it's all good.

HIS

Being Dominated

Because men are still in large part expected to be the initiators when it comes to sex, it's understandable that giving up this control and submitting completely to a woman is a very common fantasy. Whether it's being told how hard to lick or lying back and letting you do whatever you want to him, what's not to like?

Being Tied Up

Maybe it brings out the cowboy in him when you lasso him. Having his hands and feet tied to the bed while you tease him with your breasts, hands, and mouth can be excruciatingly lovely.

Getting Spanked

While the fantasy of getting spanked obviously relates to the idea of giving up control, there's something especially vulnerable about a grown man getting his naked bum spanked that says "I've been such a bad boy. Please punish me. I deserve it."

Watching

It is often said that men are visual creatures. And most of them grow up watching porn. So it's no surprise that the idea of catching a glimpse of real live nakedness, especially real live nakedness that's engaged in some sort of sexual act, is a big turn-on.

Being Watched

If he's expected to make a performance of it, he might as well have an audience. Plus, why should women get all the attention? He wants to know what it feels like to be sexually objectified.

Threesomes

While men don't seem to fantasize as much about being with another man as women do about being with another woman (at least they're not admitting it as often), many guys love the idea of being with you and another woman.

Anal Penetration

Despite the good front, more guys are curious about anal penetration than they would like to admit. The excitement stems from a curiosity about what it feels like to be penetrated (again, why should girls get all the fun?) as well as from the taboo surrounding anal sex in our culture, especially for men.

- -

Quick Tip: Just Say It

If you're nervous about bringing up a sexual concern or need, think about why. What's the worst that can happen? What if you do hurt her feelings? Yes, it's a risk, but even if something doesn't come out quite right, you can do a lot of damage control with a heartfelt apology and some explanation. Are you afraid that if you suggest something he might not want to do it or it might freak him out? Well, unlikely, but if that happens, you might need to have a discussion outside of bed to talk about being more open-minded about each other's desires and needs. Or he might actually appreciate the guidance, do what you want, maybe even see it as an invitation to offer you some insight as to what he'd like—and you'll end up with more satisfying sex. Bingo.

- -

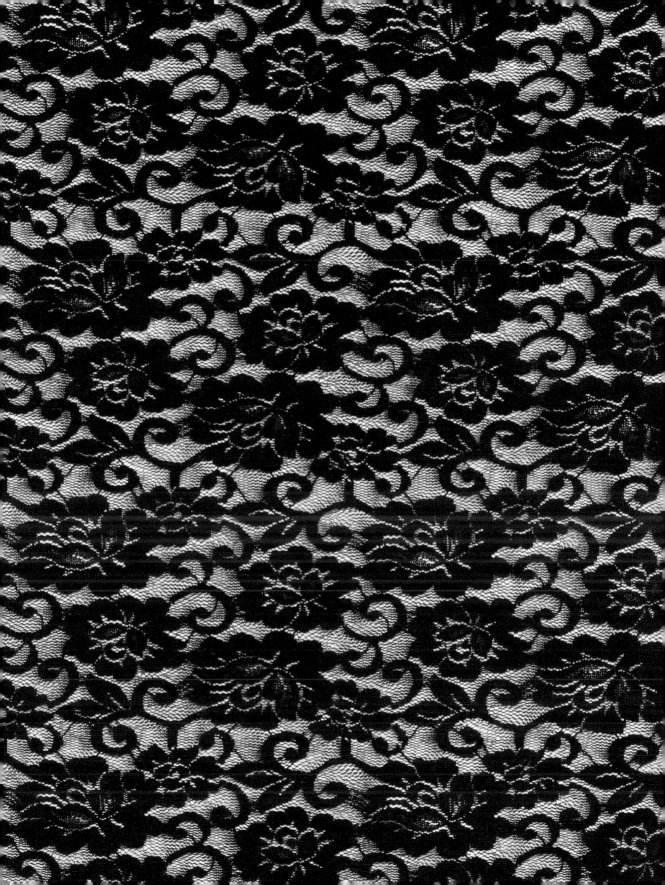

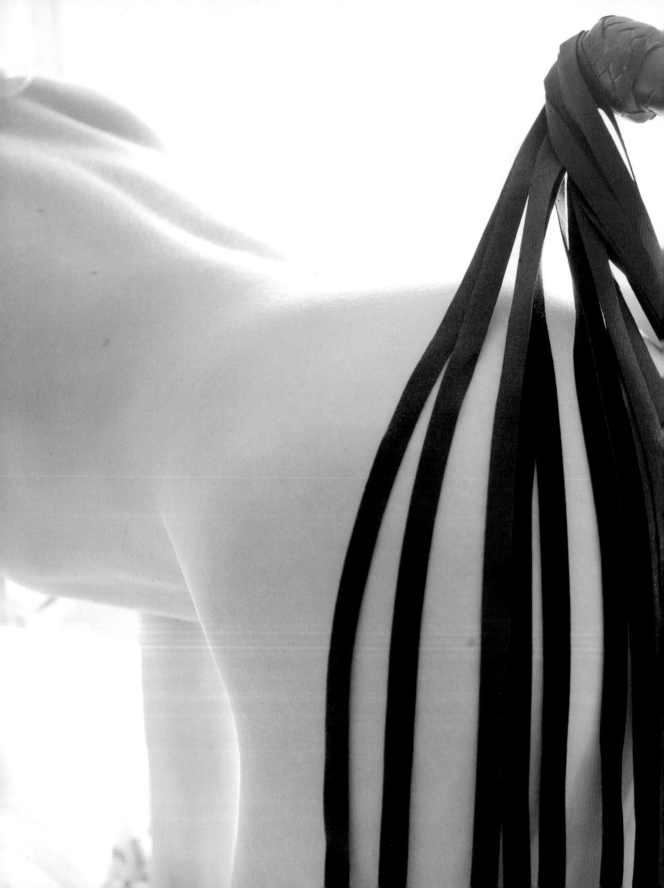

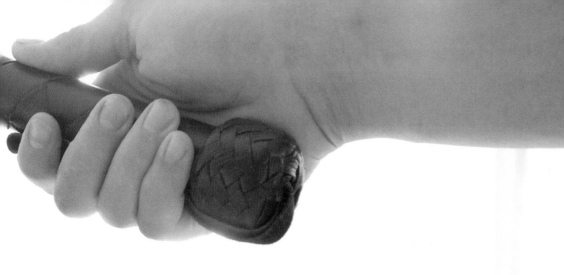

Chapter Fourteen
KINK

Have you ever held her wrists above her head during intercourse? Have you ever bit into his shoulder or felt the urge to give his butt a spank during sex? Just because you don't have a supply of floggers and ball gags in your house doesn't mean you don't have a kinky side that wants to come out and play once in a while. Don't worry, opening the door to a little kinky play doesn't mean you'll never want to leave again or that you'll need more and more extreme kicks to keep it interesting. Fuzzy handcuffs are not a gateway drug. Who knows, maybe you will discover that kink is totally your thing and eventually find yourself skipping off handcuffed hand in handcuffed hand to the nearest fetish club. But ultimately, the two of you are in control and get to decide at all times how far things will go. That's the beauty of being an adult sexual being.

If this is new territory for the two of you, I'm sure you have a few questions. Like, what exactly is kink, anyway? For the uninitiated, "kink" is just a more general term for BDSM. As I mentioned earlier, this abbreviation includes several elements: The "B" of BDSM stands for bondage, which can mean anything from tying your partner to the bed to hog-tying them suspended from the ceiling using elaborate Japanese rope techniques. "D" stands for discipline, anything from a light spanking to a full bull-whipping. "D" also stands for dominance and pairs with "S," submission. While this may conjure up images of a leather-clad mistress admonishing the hooded and ball-gagged slave kneeling at her feet, it's really just a more complex way of describing the power dynamic you can create when one of you is in control of the play—the dominant or top—and the other is submissive—the bottom. The "S" in BDSM also does double duty by standing for sadism, named for the sexually sadistic master of them all, the Marquis de Sade, an eighteenth-century (that's right, this whole kink thing isn't exactly new) French aristocrat, writer and all-around kinky guy. A sadist derives pleasure from administering pain, while the "M" in BDSM stands for masochism, that is, the enjoyment of pain, making a masochist the perfect partner for Mr. or Mrs. Sadist. Yay, everyone's happy.

But what's so sexy about administering pain or getting hurt, especially with the person you supposedly love, you ask? Well, for one, we're not talking about the kind of pain you feel when, say, you slam your hand in the car door. When combined with pleasurable sensations—imagine him running a feather across your nipple and playfully pinching it immediately after—a little bit of pain can feel glorious. It releases feel-good endorphins, takes you out of your head and puts you in touch with pure sensation. This, combined with your trust that he would never let any real harm come to you, can tap into a very deep part of your sexual psyche.

Quick Tip: Play Safe

BDSM practitioners use something called a "safe word" to stop any play they aren't comfortable with, either physically or mentally. For hardcore BDSMers, "stop" doesn't necessarily work because overriding their partner's pleas to stop may be a previously agreed-upon part of the play. Instead they use words like "red" for stop, "yellow" for slow down and "green" for full speed ahead. If you're just dabbling, agreeing to stop when your partner says "Stop" or "Slow down, wait a sec, my pubic hair's caught in the rope" will probably suffice.

Pushing yourselves outside of your usual comfort zone can be an emotional and physical thrill that allows you to explore pleasure you've never known, to add a whole other layer of adventure and possibility to your sex life, and to deepen your trust, your communication, your intimacy and ultimately, your connection as a couple.

TIME to PLAY

Five Minutes or Less

That Tickles

Bring out your inner bratty big brother. Wrestle her to the floor, straddle her and tickle her until she begs for mercy. As she's fighting to get away, lean over and French kiss her.

A Quick Tweak

Several seconds into a deep, passionate kiss, reach down and grab his nipple between your thumb and forefinger, twisting it (gently, but not too gently) as you squeeze, and intensify your kiss.

Blind Taste Test

Kink is all about awakening your senses, which doesn't always have to include pain. Tease her taste buds and explore a sweeter side of kink by making tonight's dessert more interesting. After the main course, tie a silk scarf around her eyes or slip a blindfold on her and feed her a bowl of cool, creamy ice cream or a plate of delicious, juicy fruit. Ask her to describe the tastes and sensations in her mouth with as much detail as possible. Intersperse each spoonful with a warm, wet kiss.

AT YOUR FINGERTIPS

Blindfold or silk scarf

Ice cream, fresh fruit or both

One Hour or Less

A Simple Slap

Incorporate a little pain into your regular pleasure and see how you both like it. No need to bring out the paddles or heavy artillery. Simply give her bum a swat while you're entering her from behind, or give his rear a few spanks as he is coming inside of you. Besides being sexy to look at, bums are great for spanking because they're nicely padded to help cushion the blows. Spanking can literally turn up the heat by getting the blood flowing to the area. And with the bum located right next door to the genitals, the potential to combine pain with pleasure is conveniently all in one location.

Take Control

This is a great exercise if you have a hard time giving him direction during sex (or vice versa). Sometimes it's easier to speak up when you're explicitly asking him to do something as part of a role. No need to dress up or anything. Simply "bossing" him through the sex you normally have can be kinky. Sure, you both love it when you're on top, but what's it like when you're calling the shots every step of the way? Let him caress your breasts one thrust and then forbid him from touching you the next thrust. Hover your hot stuff over his shuddering staff until he's begging you to lower yourself onto him, then make him wait even longer. Keep the game going as long as you are both comfortable and enjoying it. Remember that while, yes, you're the boss of him, you want to be a kind and compassionate boss rather than a mean boss who might say things you regret later. If either one of you gets uncomfortable, stop the game immediately (if you have a safe word, this would be the time to use it), so that no one gets hurt either physically or emotionally.

Don't Turn Me Loose

Experiment with restraint during sex. Pin her wrists to the bed with your hands while you enter her in the missionary position. Use a belt or some cotton rope to bind her wrists together over her head and attach them to the bed so she can't use them while you give her mind-blowing oral sex. Tie his hands and feet to a chair and do a strip tease in front of him. Make sure it includes some lap grinding just to make him really crazy.

All Night
A Good Spanking

If you've both discovered that you quite enjoy getting smacked on the butt during sex, you may want to spend an entire evening exploring the world of spanking further. Text him at work and tell him that you're very disappointed that he left his dishes in the sink this morning and that you plan to give him a good spanking when you get home. Then follow up on your threat.

AT YOUR FINGERTIPS

Spanking instrument
(hand, paddle, leather belt, riding crop)

Ice

Lube

Here are some ideas and guidelines for a naughty night of discipline:

Get into Position

You can spank your partner as she lies on her tummy on the bed or across your lap. Having him on all fours or bending over the back of a couch also works.

Choose Your Instrument

The good thing about using your hands to spank is that the skin-to-skin contact offers natural biofeedback so you'll have a good sense of how hard you're spanking.

A cupped hand stings less than a flat hand and makes a better smacking sound, which can add to the sexual excitement. You can also use the back of a hairbrush, a leather belt or a specially designed spanking paddle purchased from a sex shop.

Get into the Spirit

Role-play sometimes makes it easier to get into spanking. Even simple talk about how your partner has been bad and must be disciplined, while cliché, can do the trick. Go with it and really ham it up. This is supposed to be fun and playful, remember.

Build the Heat

Warm up your partner's bottom first with some gentle cheek rubbing, pinching and squeezing. This not only feels nice but will prepare the bum for what's to come by getting the blood flowing and the endorphins (the body's built-in temporary painkillers) pumping.

Ramp Up the Intensity

Whether you are using a paddle specifically designed for spanking, the back of a hairbrush or your bare hands, start slow and work your way up to greater intensity. Talk about what you're going to do before you do it to build anticipation. Or don't. Not knowing when the next spank is coming can also build excitement. The more sexually aroused she is, the more intensity she'll be able to take. As the intensity increases, the brain releases endorphins that raise her pain threshold. Combining pushing the pain threshold with a soft skin caress or a brush of your fingers across her clitoris will have her balancing on the deliciously fine line between pain and pleasure. Restrict your blows to the fleshy part of the bum where the large glute muscles can absorb more impact. If you spank too high up on the bum toward the lower back, you can get dangerously close to the kidneys, which don't enjoy the spanking so much.

Alternate Sensations

Follow a more intense smack with some lovely circular bum caresses. Cool off a red bum with some ice.

Add Genital Touch

As you're both getting into it, let your hand slide between her legs every few spanks and brush across her vulva. Slide a wet (use some lube if she's not wet) finger up and down her clitoris and into her vagina once or twice before going back to spanking. If you're spanking him, circle your other hand around the base of his genitals and tug gently between spanks. Or stroke his penis up and down a few times.

Going All the Way

Spanking can be used as an opening act to intercourse or other sexual play, or it can be an act all on its own. If you want to bring her to orgasm, you may find that spanking alone is enough of a turn-on to get her off. If not, using your fingers or a vibrator on her clitoris while smacking her bum will most certainly do the trick. If you're spanking him, you can stroke his penis to orgasm or have him masturbate to orgasm while you discipline him for being such a naughty boy.

Fit to Be Tied

That time you held his wrists down while you straddled him left you breathless. When he tied your hands behind your head and then went down on you, you experienced one of the most intense orgasms you've ever had. Sound familiar? I suspect that you, my dear, have a little thing for bondage. Do you like the idea of having him at your mercy and making him submit to whatever pleasures you decide to bestow upon him? There is no denying the sexual power in knowing that you have control and can do anything you want to him, within reason and his comfort level, of course. When it comes to any kind of bondage play, safety, trust and communication are an absolute must.

If he's game for it, why not investigate this new-found interest with an evening (or afternoon, if that's more convenient) of restraint? Before you get started, you must first think about how you'd like to truss up your man. Handcuffs are often the first thing inexperienced couples buy to experiment with bondage, but bare metal handcuffs can cut in and cause pain. If you're attached to the idea of handcuffs, at least get yourself a fuzzy or fabric-covered pair. Imagine how sexy he'd look in a pair of fluffy pink handcuffs. An old pair of stockings or a satin scarf might seem tempting, but as he's wriggling around, these fabrics can really tighten and risk cutting off circulation. Not fun. Belts, neckties and even extension cords are better choices if you're looking to use something that's already lying around the house.

Quick Tip:
Confidence Builder

If you're not comfortable asking for what you want and need in other areas of your relationship, it's going to be extra hard asking for it in bed. Try asserting yourself in small ways outside the bedroom to help build your confidence. "Make me a grilled cheese sandwich—now!"

Whatever you're using to tie up your partner, you want to make it tight enough so he can't escape but not so tight it cuts off circulation. You should be able to slip two fingers between the rope—or whatever restraint you're using—and his wrist or ankle. If you want to splurge, you can buy commercial bondage kits that come with wrist and ankle cuffs. Or, if restraint is something you discover you both enjoy, invest in what most serious bondage play folk recommend: soft cotton rope. In fact, some cotton rope and a knot-tying guide in his Christmas stocking might be a nice way to introduce the idea of experimenting with bondage. Also, it's a good plan to always keep scissors handy in case your partner wants out . . . right now!

AT YOUR FINGERTIPS

Bondage material
(fluffy handcuffs, cotton rope, ankle cuffs)

Blindfold

Satin or silky fabric

Feather

Lube

Vibrator

Once you've figured out how you're going to tie him up, you have to decide where to tie him up. If you have bedposts, tying his wrists and ankles to them is the easiest way to go. If you're serious and want to invest some money in your new hobby, you can buy sheets with built-in ankle and wrist cuffs. If you don't have bedposts and can't find another way to attach him to your bed, tie his wrists and feet to a chair. Now that he's at your mercy, you have the pleasure of electing what to do with him. I've got a few ideas:

• Let your hands and fingers travel over his entire body. Nibble his neck, tweak his nipples or stimulate his genitals while he squirms about in that glorious space between agony and pleasure.

• Keep him further on edge by interspersing all this wonderful touch and sensation with a little pain. A long, slow scratch across his penis, followed by a soft caress, for example. Take his penis deep in your mouth for a few seconds and then pinch his nipple.

• Tease him with your voice. Tell him how excited it makes you seeing him like this. Let him know how much you are enjoying yourself and how turned on you are to see him so aroused.

• What you don't touch is almost more important than what you do touch. He may be dying for you to touch his penis and, because his hands are tied, he can't touch it himself, so the longer you deny him the crazier you'll drive him. Give him a taste by very briefly brushing the flat palm of your hand along his erect penis. This will build his excitement even more.

• Take things up a notch by blindfolding him using either a scarf or a commercial blindfold. Now you've limited his ability to touch and to see. This will heighten his other senses, and not knowing what you're going to do next will get him even more excited.

• While he waits in anticipation, walk around the house and grab any textured items you can find—a (clean) scrub brush, a feather duster, silk underwear—and brush them across his body. Get him to try to identify each item. Or just have him lie back and bask in the various sensations and the excitement of not knowing what's coming next.

• While you can certainly have a ton of fun teasing him and taking him to the edge of orgasm (or over, if you choose to) using sensation, touch, oral pleasure and toys, having intercourse while he is tied up would no doubt be the cherry on the sundae for him. Whether he's lying back or sitting in a chair, climb aboard and let him enjoy the show. You can grind yourself into him and completely control the speed and depth of penetration while he surrenders himself completely to you.

• If he's tied to the bed, cover his body and face with an old sheet into which you've cut strategic holes for his nipples and jewels. Tease him through these openings while he can't see what's going on. Dance a feather or a crop-style tickler (a fringe of long rubber tails on a wand, available in most sex shops) lightly across his penis and across his nipples. Squeeze some lube into your hand and stroke his penis. If he starts to tense up like he might come, pull away before he can. Once his orgasm subsides, start stroking again. See how long you can keep it up before you grant the poor guy release.

I Am Too the Boss of You

Tonight, discover your inner dominatrix. Put on a leather jacket and some high-heeled boots to help with the psychological transformation. Or, if you really want to get into character, visit a sex shop and get yourself an entire dominatrix ensemble, complete with knee-high spike-heeled boots, stockings, garters, a leather or PVC bustier and a whip. The more you dress up for the part, the more it will help you to get out of your own head and play the role.

- -

Quick Tip:
Take Control

If you're usually submissive, try out a dominant relationship in your role-play, like boss/employee or drill sergeant/cadet.

- -

Once you're decked out, work on discovering and getting comfortable with your sexy, bossy voice. Start with simple, non-sexual orders. Boss him around the house. Command him to do the dishes or whatever chores need to be done. Supervise to make sure he's doing them right. Scold him if he isn't and make him do them again. Once you feel confidently in character, take it to the bedroom. Tell him how you want him to undress and correct him if he doesn't do something exactly as you instruct.

AT YOUR FINGERTIPS

High-heeled boots

Garter and stockings

Leather or PVC bustier or jacket

Whip

Use your control every step of the way. Instruct him on how you would like him to pleasure you. Each time he does something right, reward him—a few strokes of his manhood, a deep kiss, nothing too elaborate. Then turn the attention back to you. Tell him he must lick your nipples for exactly three minutes without coming up for air. When he does something you don't like, voice your disapproval and make him do it again until he does it exactly the way you want him to. Keep the play going as long as you're both enjoying it. In fact, why restrict your role to one night of sexual fun? Be the boss of him for the whole weekend and see where it takes you.

❧Spice Cheat Sheet❧

☐ Text your sweetie a sexy fantasy in ten words or less.

☐ Wrestle her to the floor, straddle her and tickle her until she begs for mercy.

☐ Go to a sex shop together and explore the costume section.

☐ Squeeze his nipple hard while you deep-kiss him.

☐ Surf for fantasy erotica on the Internet and find a few sexy stories you can read to each other.

☐ Download some porn and watch it together. She picks.

☐ Put your hair in a bun, don some glasses and "teach" him how to pleasure you.

☐ Surf the adult classifieds together and pick potential threesome partners.

☐ The next time you're having sex doggie-style, tell her she's been a naughty girl and give her a few spanks on the bottom.

☐ Play dominatrix tonight and tell him exactly what you want him to do to please you.

☐ Tie him to the bed blindfolded so you can tickle his naked body with objects you've gathered around the house.

☐ Establish a safe word that will stop play immediately.

TIME TO GO

Remember what I told you at the beginning of this book? We make time for the things we *want* or *desire*. If you don't have time for sex, some part of you has lost some of that desire. How do you eat an elephant? One bite at a time. How do you create more desire in your relationship? One sexy ear nibble at a time.

You need to work every day to make each other feel cherished, loved, sexy, appreciated and desirable. But it doesn't have to take a lot of time. I hope I've inspired you with lots of ideas that take mere seconds to mere minutes a day. While some of them may feel awkward and forced at first, the positive response you get from your partner will motivate and encourage you. This in turn will make you want to do more things to stir your partner's desire.

I hope this book has made you realize that while you may feel like there is no time for sex in your busy schedule, in fact, there is. It may be a challenge to carve out the time for a long, romantic night of lovemaking, but hey, throwing her onto the bed for a hot quickie before you go out tonight counts as sex too. And sex doesn't always have to be intercourse. Sex can be everything from a teasing fondle under the table to a full evening of sexual role-play, complete with costumes.

Connect in sexual ways each day. Take five seconds to compliment her or ten seconds to kiss him deeply, give him a five-minute morning blow job or spend an hour to go sex toy shopping instead of kids' toys shopping together, and I guarantee that the two of you will be having better sex . . . in no time.

⚛ Make a Plan ⚛

I'm going to leave you and your partner with one last exercise that will help you get the most out of this book and give you a game plan for your sex life during the next weeks, months, even years. Do this exercise separately. Grab a pen and a piece of paper and sit down with this book. Flip through each section and write down any activities you come across that you'd like to try. Be as thorough or as brief as you like. You can always add to your list later. Some evening after you've both made your lists, pour a couple of glasses of wine, sit down together and compare. Mark yes, no or maybe beside each item on your partner's list to indicate your comfort level with that activity. Now you've got a game plan. Activities with a yes from both of you go into the "to do" pile, maybes go into the "to be discussed" pile, and nos get tossed, at least for now. You can always redraft your lists if things change down the road. Have fun!

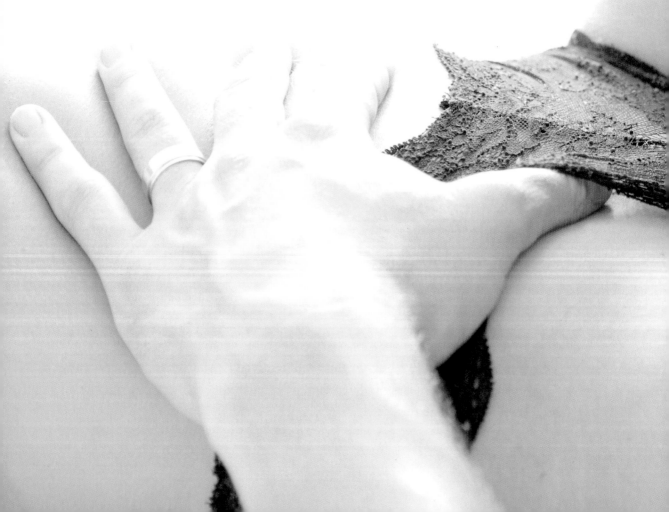

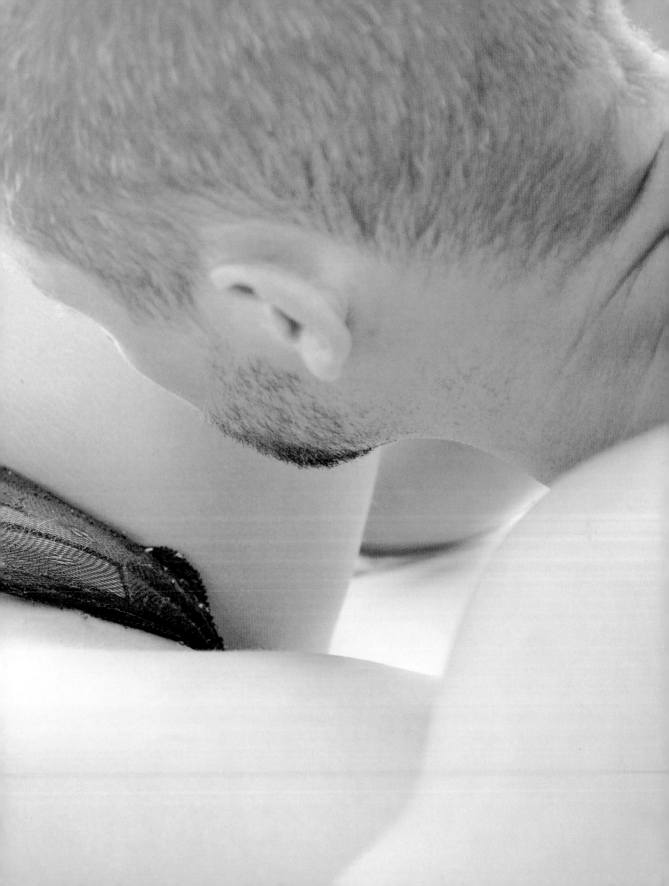

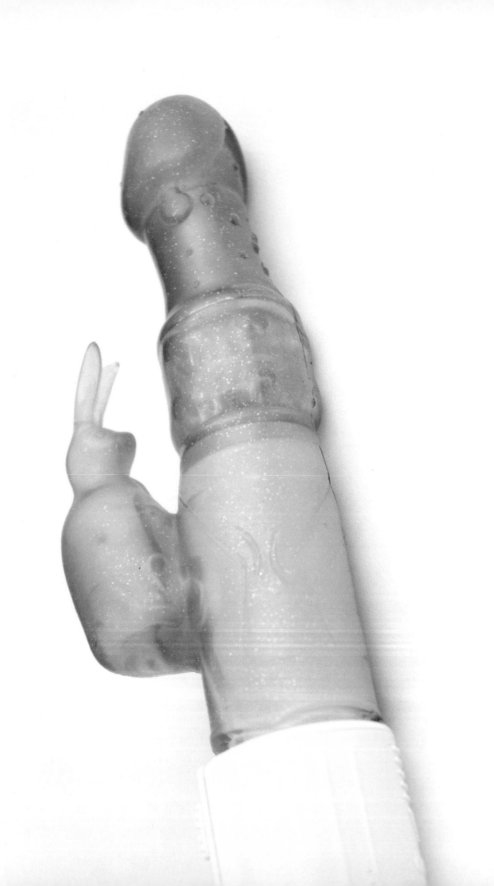

Appendix A
Toys

Thanks to **Good for Her** (goodforher.com) for generously providing the toys for the photos shown here.

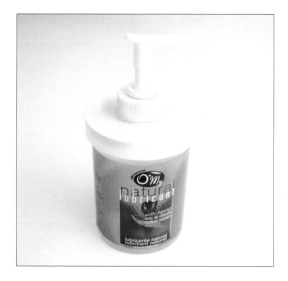

LUBE

Lubricant isn't technically a toy, but it's the easiest, cheapest and most effective single thing you can buy to enhance your sex life. Whether it comes in a plastic pump bottle or a hand-blown Italian glass bottle (yes, lubes are getting quite classy these days), lube makes sex more slippery and exciting. It improves solo or mutual masturbation, toy play, intercourse, anal sex and anything in between. Even if you use lubricated condoms, try adding a drip of lube inside the tip to increase his pleasure and reduce the chance of breakage.

The lube market has come a long way since K-Y Jelly (even K-Y Jelly has come a long way since the original K-Y Jelly) with lubes that warm, tingle, taste and do windows (okay, I'm pretty sure lube would do a lousy job on your windows). Parabens are preservatives often used in commercial lubricants (as well as many cosmetics and fragrances), and while the jury is still out on this, some research has shown them to be carcinogenic. If this concerns you, look for organically sourced, preservative-free massage oils and lubricants. There is conflicting information out there about whether the glycerin used to sweeten most flavoured lubricant encourages the growth of yeast, so if you are a woman who is prone to yeast infections, you may want to stick to glycerin-free lube just to be on the safe side. Check a brand's website or ask the salesperson if you want to verify the ingredients.

Most lubes are available in trial samples that you can pick up for a buck or two, so you can test drive a variety until you find one or a few you like. Whatever the added bells and whistles, all lubes can be divided into the following three categories:

Water-Based

Pros: Relatively inexpensive, widely available and can be used with toys made of any material. It is also safe to use with condoms, washes off easily with warm water, and comes in warming, tingling and flavoured varieties.

Cons: Dries up more quickly. Keep a glass of water by the bed so you can dip your fingers and add water to the lube to reactivate it.

Silicone-Based

Pros: Doesn't contain water and therefore doesn't dry up as quickly. Stays on in water and doesn't absorb into the skin. Can be used with condoms. A little goes a long way. *Cons:* Pricier (but you use less). Needs to be washed off with soap and water. Will damage any toys containing silicone.

Oil-Based

Pros: Inexpensive (baby oil will do). Doesn't dry up and is less sticky than water-based or silicone lube.

Cons: Breaks down latex condoms or toys.

SEX TOYS 101

Sex toys add a whole new dimension to your sex life. They can facilitate communication (you can't just haul out a glow-in-the-dark dildo without first having at least a quick chat). They bring an element of playfulness to your relationship (there's a reason they're called "toys"). They up the pleasure by introducing new sensations and encouraging experimentation. Finally, for our purposes here, when time is at a premium, toys can help get you where you both want to go faster and with less effort.

Given the size and scope of the sex toy market and, quite honestly, the amount of crap available out there, you want to be a well-informed shopper so you don't waste your hard-earned money. Unfortunately, for years the sex toy industry has been able to get away with selling people junk simply because most people are so embarrassed to even be seen in a sex shop that they'll slap their money down on anything just to get the heck out of there.

Thankfully, the industry is changing and there are lots of fantastic new toy manufacturers, designers and developers who actually seem to give a hoot about the quality of people's sexual experiences. And in the last decade or so a whole crop of friendly, urban sex shops have popped up that are a far cry from the old seedy shop with the creepy blow-up doll in the window. These new shops often have well-informed, sex-positive staff who make toy shopping a bit like shoe shopping, helping you find the right style, fit and comfort level. Some even serve tea!

Still, it's easy to be overwhelmed by the vast array of products out there. Arming yourself with some general info on materials, models, quality and safety will save you time and stress when shopping. But before you rev up your shopping cart, let's first take a minute or two to dispel three misconceptions many people have:

They're Just for the Ladies

Ever since *Sex and the City* turned the Rabbit Pearl vibrator into an instant celebrity and made sex toys as obligatory an accessory as the latest "It" bag, it seems no woman's bedside table is expected to be without one . . . or two . . . or six. But sex toys are not an exclusively female bedside accessory. More and more toys for boys and couples are showing up on the market. So get over the idea that sex toys are meant for a lonely single woman curled up with her battery-operated date on a Saturday night (though add a sexy movie, some lube and some satin sheets and it doesn't sound all that bad).

They're Addictive

People who are freaked out about the idea of sex toys often argue that once you start using them you won't be able to have sex without them. This is simply not true. Just because a woman learns to orgasm using a vibrator doesn't mean she won't be able to come any other way. In fact, I would argue the opposite is true. Sex toys can help you learn about your sexual response and the type of stimulation, pressure and movement you need to get off. Obviously

anything done to excess isn't healthy. So if you're at the point where you're calling in sick so you can stay home and play with your vibrator all day, you might want to back off a little.

They Replace the Real Thing

Perhaps, as a guy, you're concerned that a vibrator will put you out of business and your woman will ride off into the sunset on her Hitachi Magic Wand. Or that you're a "bad lover" because you can't get her off on your own. Rest easy. Vibrators are not a substitute for the Real Thing, they're a "thing" in themselves. They are simply fun tools that can provide enhancement and assistance. Rather than treat them as a rival, embrace them and the fun they can bring to your sex life. And consider all the wear and tear they can save on your tongue and fingers!

HOW TO CHOOSE A TOY

Okay, assumptions dispelled, you're both keen to explore the world of toys. Here are some basic guidelines to get you started:

Find a Shop You Like

As mentioned, you no longer need to don a trench coat to visit your local sex store. Most large cities have sex shops that are couple- and female-friendly, with informed and open-minded staff members who make it easy to ask even the most delicate questions. If you don't have a shop like this near you, most of these stores have websites that allow you to buy online and order from the comfort of your own home.

Be Sensitive

If you shop in an actual store, stick close to one another and pay attention to what items draw your partner's attention and what makes them uncomfortable.

What Do You Want to Do with It?

Do you want a toy for external use, penetration or both? If you want a good buzz and don't necessarily want penetration, egg-shaped vibrators are great. Dildos or phallic-shaped vibrators are best for penetration, while multi-purpose vibrators offer both penetration and external vibration.

Consider How Powerful a Toy You Need

If you're a woman who can climax from manual stimulation or is easily orgasmic, you'll be fine with a model that takes two AA batteries. If orgasm is more difficult for you, you might consider something stronger or even a plug-in. Plastic toys create a more intense vibration, while the vibration from rubber or silicone toys is more diffused.

What Do You Want It to Look Like?

Personally, I'm not a big fan of toys that look like real sex organs. They creep me out. The lifelike look might work for you, but if not, there are many beautifully designed toys on the market today that come in plenty of fun colours and interesting shapes.

Pick a Material

Toys made of 100 percent silicone and elastomers are better quality but usually more expensive, whereas hard plastic toys are cheaper. Rubber and latex toys may cause an allergic reaction.

Start Simple

Begin with a simple, inexpensive toy—$20 to $30—to see if you both even like using a toy before you shell out big bucks for something more fancy and durable.

SEX TOY SAFETY

When it comes to safety and sex toys, there's the obvious stuff. Unless you want to end up as one of the "sex toy retrieval cases" an emergency doctor friend of mine assures me he sees on an alarmingly regular basis, never insert anything that won't be easy to extract. In other words, what goes up must come down.

Unfortunately, there isn't a lot of research on the safety of sex toys or the materials used to make them, though this is starting to change as sex toys become more popular. Until more reliable information becomes available, there are a few red flags you should heed:

"Novelty Purposes Only"

Any product with this warning on the package is best avoided unless you want a gag gift for a bridal shower. Basically, this is a catch-all phrase commonly used in the sex toy industry to protect companies from liability when the product is manufactured to a substandard quality with unsafe materials.

Hoaxes

If the pitch for a lotion or potion sounds like a hoax, it probably is. Anything that promises to make your penis grow, your boobs bigger, your orgasm better or your erection harder or longer lasting is bogus.

Latex

Some people are sensitive or even allergic to latex and break out in a rash if they use latex condoms or latex gloves. If you have a reaction to latex, it's important to realize that sex toys may also have latex in them. Unfortunately, because manufacturers aren't required to list the materials in their toys, it's difficult to know for sure if a rubber-based

toy contains latex. Stick to plastic, acrylic or even metal toys; if you want a toy made out of a softer, more pliable material, 100 percent silicone toys made by a reputable company are your best bet.

Phthalates

These chemicals—pronounced "thal-ates"—soften rubber and have been used since the 1920s in everything from kids' toys to medical instruments, pesticides and, yes, sex toys. Much debate has arisen in recent years as to their safety, and an increasing body of research suggests the stuff is toxic (it's been linked to cancer and reproductive organ damage in rats). For now, do some research and decide on your comfort level or simply choose phthalate-free toys made from hard plastic, glass, metal, 100 percent silicone or elastomer.

SEX TOY MATERIALS

Sex toys are made from a variety of materials, all of which have their pros and cons. Here's a guide to the most common:

Rubber or Jelly

You'll recognize these toys because they feel squishy and, well, jelly-like, and are usually cheaper. Rubber and jelly are very porous materials and can be difficult to keep clean, even with soap and water. Using these toys with a condom can help keep them clean. These materials also tend to "off-gas," leaving oily stains and/or fusing to whatever they're lying against in the drawer or wherever you store them. I know, sexy, hey?

Plastic

Toys made of plastic are usually hard and smooth, like that "personal massager" you first saw in the Sears catalogue as a teenager back in the eighties. The great thing about plastic is that it is non-porous and therefore easy to clean with soap and water (just be careful not to get the battery part wet if it's a battery-operated toy). Plastic toys are also phthalate-free if that's a concern. Because they are hard, they are obviously less flexible, which can be either a pro or a con, depending on how you're using the toy. Plastic toys are usually less expensive, though this means they are often cheaply made and less durable.

Silicone

Denser than jelly or rubber toys, silicone toys are not as hard and inflexible as plastic ones. Silicone is hypoallergenic, phthalate-free, non-porous, easy to clean (you can even boil it or throw it in the dishwasher!) and durable. As a result, silicone toys are generally more expensive. But buyer beware: A toy doesn't have to be 100 percent silicone to be advertised as a silicone toy. You may be getting a rubber/silicone mix. Read the package carefully or ask the salesperson if you are unsure. Also, never use a silicone lubricant with a silicone toy because the lube will break down the material.

Elastomer

This is one of the newest sex-toy materials on the market. Slightly softer and more porous than silicone, elastomer has the flexibility and softness of rubber but is durable, hypoallergenic, and latex- and phthalate-free. Elastomer toys are more expensive and, because they are slightly porous, you may want to use a condom with them to keep them clean.

Cyberskin

This material is designed to simulate the suppleness of human skin, so it is squishy, soft and pliable. Like human skin, it is also very porous and can tear easily and therefore must be handled with care. It can be washed with soap and water, but you need to powder it with cornstarch afterward so it doesn't get sticky during storage. It should only be used with water-based lubes because silicone or oil will break down the material. Cyberskin is comparable in price to silicone or elastomer.

Acrylic, Glass, or Metal

Toys made of acrylic, glass or metal are rigid but extremely durable and smooth. Most glass toys are made of Pyrex and will not shatter even if dropped. It's a good idea to check for cracks regularly, just to be safe. Glass can be boiled clean. Metal and acrylic are shatter-free and harder to break. Many toys made of these materials are expensive but often quite beautiful and sculptural in design. Sex toys as art!

TOY CATALOGUE

Whether you want to bust the bank and shell out $325 for a 24-karat-gold water-resistant vibrator designed by Herman Miller or a $20 vibrating silver bullet, there's a toy for every budget. Here's a round-up of what's out there:

VIBRATORS
Plug-In Vibrators

The most famous of all plug-in vibrators is the Hitachi Magic Wand (below), sometimes referred to as the "Cadillac of vibrators."

Pros: Powerful, steady vibration. Unless there is a power outage, a plug-in won't let you down at that crucial moment.

Cons: Pricier than battery-operated models. Can be loud and bulky and is generally designed for external genital vibration only (though most come with attachments that can be used for penetration or other types of stimulation). The vibration may be too intense for some women, though you can use it through fabric to diffuse the intensity. Must be near a plug to operate so you can't walk around the house using it.

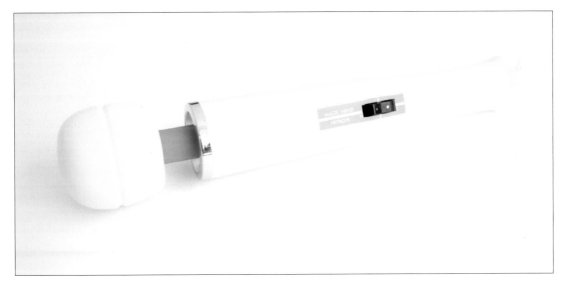

Battery-Operated Vibrators

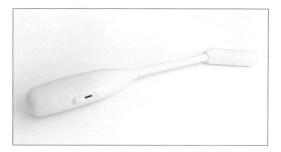

With these models, batteries are inserted directly into the vibe or into a battery pack attached to the vibe with a cord.

Pros: A wide variety of models is available at every price point, from a $10 vibrating egg to the Rabbit Pearl vibe made famous by *Sex and the City.* Many have multiple speed and vibration pattern settings. Because there is no cord to plug in, you're not tethered to the wall, so you can use it while chatting on the phone, surfing the Internet . . .

Cons: Batteries die (buy in bulk or invest in rechargeable batteries—better for the environment). They can also corrode, destroying the toy (to avoid this, always remove batteries between uses). Some battery-operated plastic toys can be of poorer quality and therefore less durable.

Rechargeable Vibrators

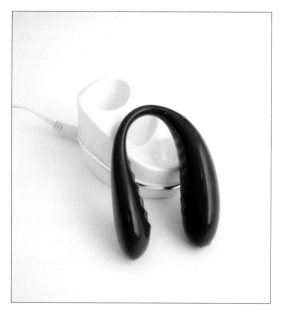

These vibes come with a plug-in adapter that allows you to recharge the toy between uses.

Pros: No need for batteries and, unlike a plug-in toy, you're not "plugged in" during use so you are less restricted in movement.

Cons: Rechargeable toys are newer to the market and often pricier than regular battery-operated toys. There's also the potential disappointment when you realize at a crucial moment that you forgot to recharge.

Solar-Powered Vibrators

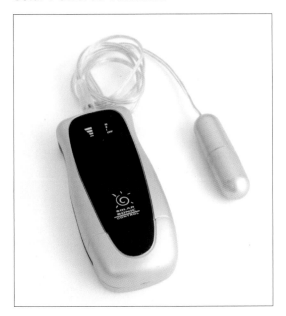

Mini Vibrators

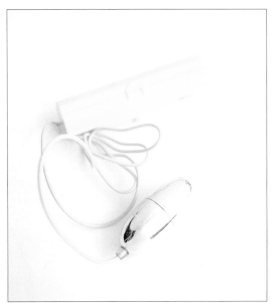

Even sex can be environmentally conscious these days. Solar-powered vibes are equipped with a small solar panel that allows you to charge it using only sunlight.

Pros: No batteries or electricity required. Great for camping or having sex on the beach!

Cons: Rainy days (and isn't that when you need it most?). Be sure to keep it charged. You'll need to keep it out where it can get enough light to charge between uses. Not so convenient when the kids jump into bed and start using it as a cellphone.

Battery-operated pocket rockets and vibrating eggs or bullets are compact, convenient and discreet. Some have a battery control pack attached by wire to the toy while others contain the battery and are switched on and controlled by twisting one end of the toy.

Pros: Because they are small and mighty and can be held by the fingertips, these allow for a lot of control and pressure by the user and can provide great clitoral stimulation during intercourse without getting in the way.

Cons: Some women find the vibration too intense (some mini vibes come with rubber sleeves to diffuse the vibration). These small toys can't be inserted vaginally or anally.

Wearable Vibrators

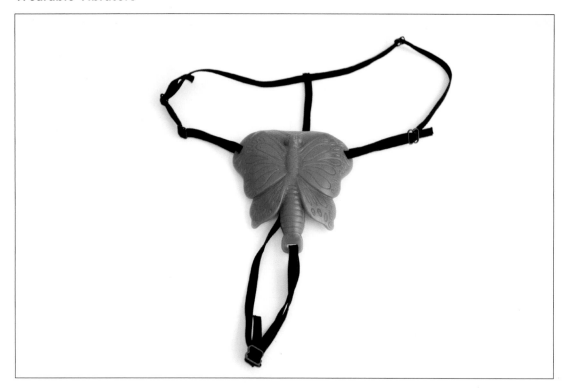

Usually in the form of a butterfly or some other creature with a mini vibe tucked inside—and straps that go around the waist and thighs so that the vibrator is positioned over her clitoral area. Newer models like the Canadian-designed We-Vibe (pictured on page 244) are designed to be worn during penetration. Shaped like an elongated C with a tiny vibrator on each end, one arm of the vibe lies over her clitoral area while the other arm is inserted and vibrates against her G spot as he penetrates her.

Pros: They can be worn during penetration or while both your hands are busy doing other things. The We-Vibe design offers simultaneous clitoral and G-spot stimulation for her as well as added vibration for him during penetration. The newest model is waterproof, rechargeable and remote controlled.

Cons: The cheaper models are usually poorly designed, and you'll need to use your hands to position the vibrator on her clitoris, undermining the whole hands-free novelty.

Finger Vibrators

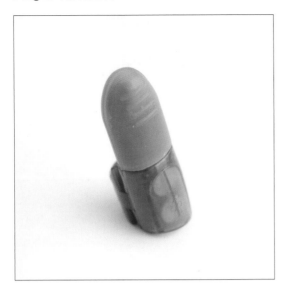

Vibrating Rings

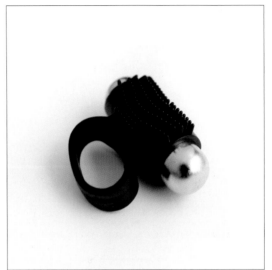

Tiny vibes that can be slipped over or clipped onto your fingertip.

Pros: Because they are small, they can be used during oral sex or intercourse without getting in the way and are comfortable and easy to control. Great for those moments when you wish your fingers could vibrate for that added extra bit of intense stimulation.

Cons: May not fit all fingers. Can cause your finger to become numb after long use. Some women may find the direct, focused stimulation too intense.

A rubber, silicone or elastomer ring with a small bullet vibrator attached to it that he wears around the base of his penis so that he feels the vibration through his penis and the vibrator hits her clitoral area as he's penetrating her. Some come with two small vibes attached, one at the top of the ring designed to hit her clitoris and one below to vibrate against his testicles.

Pros: Both partners get to enjoy vibration at the same time. Can be used during penetration without getting in the way. The tight ring around the base of his penis can help intensify his erection.

Cons: Minimal contact between the vibrator and her clitoris during intense thrusting.

Multi-Purpose or Dual Vibrators

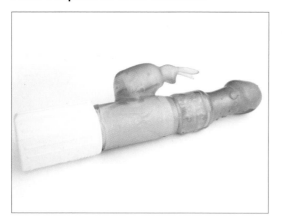

Vibrators with a long shaft for penetration as well as an extra clitoral vibrator at the base, often in the shape of a rabbit or some other little animal for some reason, like the Rabbit Pearl vibe (above). Separate controls operate each part independently.

Pros: Provide penetration and vibration at the same time. Some have "pearls" embedded partway down the shaft that swirl around at the vaginal opening when inserted.

Cons: Often pricey and not always the best quality for the money. All the bells and whistles don't necessarily pay off—for example, the clitoral vibrator often seems like an afterthought because the stimulating parts don't necessarily match up with her most sensitive lady parts.

Ergonomic Vibrators

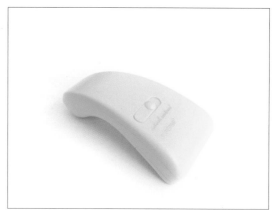

One of the newest trends in sex toys, these often beautifully designed vibrators are made to fit the contours of her body and are not necessarily designed for penetration. They are usually made of plastic or silicone.

Pros: Fit snugly against her vulva diffusing vibration into the entire area. Some women prefer the non-phallic shape. Most are designed by smaller manufacturers and tend to be well made.

Cons: These designer vibes can be quite pricey. Also, the vibrating area designed to lie over the clitoris often gives a more diffused vibration that may not provide enough direct stimulation to achieve orgasm.

G-Spot Vibrators

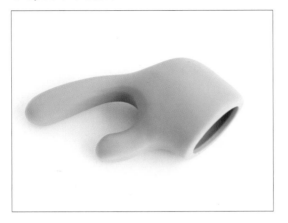

Vibrators designed to curve along the front inside wall of the vagina when inserted to stimulate the G spot. Many models of plug-in and some battery-operated vibrators come with G-spot attachments.

Pros: Using this in conjunction with fingers or a vibrator on the clitoris can sometimes result in a G-spot orgasm.

Cons: Using a G-spot vibe doesn't automatically result in ejaculation and may set up unrealistic expectations and create added pressure and frustration.

Remote-Control Vibrators

Mini vibes that usually come with a pair of underwear rigged with a pocket to hold the vibrator in place over her crotch while the operator runs the remote.

Pros: The idea of being able to literally turn her on from across the room is exciting; no cords to get tangled up in.

Cons: You might get funny looks when that strange humming sound comes out from under the table and your partner starts wiggling around in her seat (then again, that could be a pro if that's part of the fun). As with other wearable vibes, simply feeling general vibration in her genital area won't necessarily make her come.

Waterproof Vibrators

Battery-operated vibes covered in special water-resistant materials allow for extra fun in the tub or other wet venues.

Pros: Great for sex in the shower or bathtub, lake or swimming pool.

Cons: Masturbating or stimulating your partner with a rubber duck may weird you out, though since the original vibrating rubber duck appeared more models are becoming available that don't resemble cute small animals. Waterproof casing may dull vibration.

DILDOS

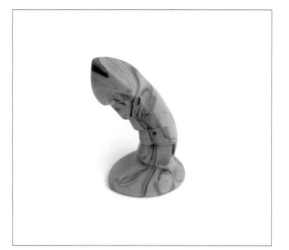

A non-vibrating, phallic-shaped sex toy used for oral, anal and vaginal penetration. Dildos can be made of rubber, latex, vinyl or silicone and come in lots of shapes and sizes. Some are curved to hit the G spot. Some are veined or ribbed to provide texture.

Pros: She can enjoy the feeling of being penetrated while masturbating. When his penis isn't available or has had its fill, a dildo can keep the fun going.

Cons: Penetration with a dildo alone may not be enough to bring her to orgasm. Some dildos are designed to fit a small bullet vibrator in the base. The vibration isn't as intense as that of a regular vibrator because it is diffused through the dildo, but it can add a lovely sensation to penetration.

HARNESSES

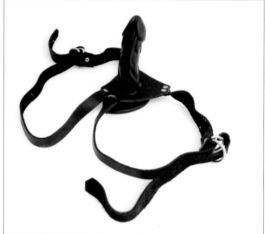

Harnesses are strapped around the waist and thighs and designed to hold a dildo so that a woman can penetrate a man anally or penetrate another woman.

Pros: Allows her to enjoy the feeling of having her own "penis" and the two of you to reverse roles.

Cons: Many commercial harnesses are poorly designed—they don't fit well or the straps cut into your flesh. Luckily, lots of smaller designers make excellent harnesses out of leather, rubber and other materials. These tend to be pricier but are definitely worth the extra cost.

ANAL TOYS

Anal Beads

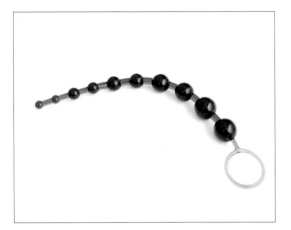

Butt Plugs

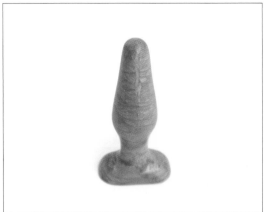

Anal beads are smooth plastic, rubber or silicone balls spaced slightly apart on a string so that the beads can be inserted or removed one at a time using the ring or handle at the end of the string. The beads are often sized from smaller to bigger so you can increase the intensity with each ball as arousal increases.

Pros: Because the beads are inserted one at a time, your partner can relax after each bead until they are ready for the next one.

Cons: Some of the cheaper plastic models may have sharp edges where the plastic is moulded together. Cotton string between beads can be hard to clean. Silicone beads are often strung together with silicone, which is easier to clean.

Butt plugs come in various materials, shapes, sizes and textures, but most are in the shape of an elongated triangle with a tapered tip and a flared base so that it can't slip all the way inside. They come thin— for beginners—and thicker for the more experienced. You can also find butt plugs that have a small egg-shaped vibrator in the base to add a vibrating sensation.

Pros: These can be inserted and left in during intercourse or other sexual activity, providing another level of stimulation.

Cons: Getting used to the feeling of holding something in your butt while doing other things takes some practice. A few projectile butt plug incidents may be unavoidable. Hey, remember, toys are meant to make things more fun and, sometimes, well, funny.

G-Spot Anal Toys for Boys

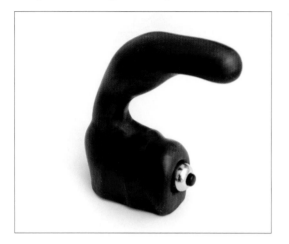

These curved, insertable phallic-shaped toys with a flared based are designed to hit and stimulate the prostate or male G spot. These toys come in vibrating and non-vibrating models.

Pros: He can use this type of toy for added stimulation during masturbation. She can use it during a hand job to stimulate his G spot, or it can be inserted and held in place during intercourse.

Cons: Some toys are quite large and, well, in this particular setting, size may very well matter.

PENIS SLEEVES

He can slide his penis into a rubber, cyberskin or elastomer sleeve for added sensation during masturbation or while she is giving him a hand job. Some sleeves vibrate and many are designed to resemble a vagina, mouth or anus. Lube it up and off you go.

Pros: Thankfully, newer designs and materials mean that penis sleeves have come a long way from the creepy plastic, hairy female "genital" models of the seventies and eighties, and the quality and variety keep getting better.

Cons: Sleeves made of softer, more pliable material like cyberskin may feel more realistic but are less durable.

COCK RINGS

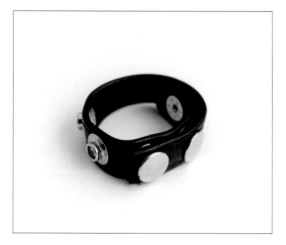

Rings made of rubber, vinyl, leather or metal are slipped over or snapped around and worn at the base of his erect penis and/or around the base of his testicles.

Pros: Can help sustain or intensify his erection by restricting blood flow out of the penis, thus allowing him to last longer. Some have tiny vibrators that can feel good for him or for both him and her if left on during intercourse.

Cons: Sometimes, a cock ring works a little too well and sustains his erection for longer than he would like, making it difficult to remove the ring. For this reason, avoid rings made out of rigid material such as metal. Use leather rings with snaps or rubber rings that can be cut off if necessary. Rubber rings can catch hairs (ouch!).

Appendix B
Troubleshooting

Sex isn't all fun and lube. The following are a few of the most common sexual issues and problems couples bring to me. So, right off the bat, if you are experiencing any of the problems listed here, you can at least take some comfort in the fact that you are definitely not alone.

COMMUNICATION

If your sexual needs are not being met, you can do one of two things: (1) stew silently and be annoyed because surely at this stage in your relationship your partner should be able to read your mind and know what you want (because just being in a relationship suddenly makes us psychic, right?), or (2) muster up a little humility and understanding and realize that the best way to get your sexual needs met is to ask for what you want. I know, crazy idea, hey? The thing is, at the beginning of most sexual relationships, when sex is new and exciting, you often don't need to talk about it. You're too busy doing it. Which means by the time you have things to talk about (and sex will inevitably become an issue in one way or another at some point in the relationship), there is no precedent. You don't know how to bring

it up. You don't know what to say. You're afraid to open a can of worms, so you both just keep the lid on and say nothing.

Many of the Quick Tips throughout this book offer advice on how to read your partner's body and how to communicate your needs and wants in specific sexual situations. But if you want to communicate about more general sexual issues and problems in your relationship, consider the following:

Is Sex the Issue?

Determine if the problem is really about sex by looking at your relationship outside of sex. Sex is a reflection and extension of the relationship. So the frustrations you're having when it comes to sex probably somehow mirror issues in the relationship. You can't fix the sex without looking at how your relationship functions. Are you getting what you want and need in other departments?

Write It Down

Before discussing a difficult sexual problem with your partner, write it down so you can clarify it in your mind before talking about it. Or talk to a friend about the problem. Hearing yourself talk about it out loud and listening to your friend's feedback can help you sort out what's going on.

Think Before You Speak

Don't be so anxious to get something out in the open and "fixed" that you don't think it through on your own first. It's a good idea to sit with an issue and wrestle with it on your own for a while before dragging your partner into it. You may find that it turns out to be something you can work through by yourself. You may find that it's about another issue entirely. Or you may find that you just had too much coffee or too little sleep that day and the problem seemed worse than it really is.

Keep Your Heart Open

This is tricky stuff: Egos and hearts are delicate. Tread lightly. Always remember, it takes two to tango. Share the responsibility for your problems. Be kind to each other. Badgering someone to open up and talk is more likely to achieve the opposite and shut them down. As when discussing any problems in all areas of the relationship—money, kids, whose turn it is to clean out the lint trap—don't point fingers or start any sentences with "You always . . ." Make an effort to really listen and understand each other.

Be Patient

Don't expect things to change immediately just because you've said something. Your sweetheart may need time to process what you've told them. You may have to talk about it again and again . . . and again. Just as with other issues in your relationship and your life, resolving sexual problems is an ongoing process.

Be Aware of How You Communicate

Bringing up an issue in a threatening, manipulating or controlling way begets resistance and anger. Discussing it in a loving, kind way usually gets better results.

Take a Risk

If you never ask for what you need and want either outside or inside the bedroom, not only do you not get it, you forfeit a wonderful opportunity to deepen your emotional and physical connection. If you never expose yourself, make yourself vulnerable or risk rejection and even embarrassment, you'll continue to keep each other at a safe distance and maintain the status quo. Communication, trust and intimacy only grow by taking risks with each other.

DIFFERING DESIRES

Differing levels of desire, mismatched sex drives, lopsided libidos, "Why the heck don't you ever want to have sex anymore?"—however you put it (though I don't suggest you put it that last way), the amount of sex you're (not) having is often a major source of relationship conflict. Most commonly, the person who wants sex feels rejected and ashamed of their desire, while the other person just wants the more ardent partner to back off or wants to be intimate without feeling pressured to do anything more than, say, kiss. Tension and resentment build on both sides, worsening the problem. What can you do?

Rethink What's "Normal"

Don't get hung up on whatever a survey or a new study say about how much sex everyone else is having. The only practical yardstick to determine whether you and a partner are having "enough" sex is how both of you feel about it. If you're both happy with how much sex you're having, great. If not, you need to deal with it.

Change Your Outgoing Message

If you're the one who doesn't want to have sex, ask yourself why. Listen to the answers in your head. If they are over-whelmingly negative—I'm tired, I feel fat, I don't have time, I don't have the energy, my partner doesn't know how to turn me on, I can't communicate what I like—any desire will be pretty much put out of its misery before it even has a chance to get past the starting gate in your brain. If you consciously replace those negative thoughts with positive ones—I really want to feel sexually connected to my partner,

my partner deserves my sexual attention, I want to overcome some of my sexual fears and learn how to tell my partner what I like, if we make time for sex we will feel connected and physically engaged—it will put you in a more sexually positive state of mind.

Speak Up

Take the next step and vocalize these positive thoughts. It only takes a few seconds to say, while lying in bed, "You know, I'd like us to have a better sex life. I realize that part of the reason we don't is because I fill my head with reasons not to have sex, like I'm too tired or scared to tell you what I like. I'm really trying to change those voices in my head to more positive messages because I love you and I want us to connect physically." Verbalizing this will at least make them feel like you're not entirely ignoring the issue and ultimately, them. This buys you time to dig your desire out from the rock it's been hiding under and identify the obstacles that are stopping you from wanting to have sex.

Don't Feel Bad About Not Wanting to Have Sex

Wanting to have sex is considered the norm. But whether you're a man or a woman, you shouldn't be ashamed or feel that you have to apologize for experiencing lack of desire.

Not everyone needs to unleash his or her inner vixen. You may be better at other things in the relationship. This doesn't let you off the hook; it just removes some of the pressure. As the low-desire half of the relationship, be aware that if you want to have any kind of sexual relationship with your partner, you'll probably have to work a little harder at it.

Give In

You do things you don't necessarily want to just to please your partner in other areas of your relationship, so why not with sex? As the lower-drive person, try having sex occasionally even if you don't feel like it. Hey, you don't always want to go to the gym either, but you usually feel better when you force yourself to go anyway.

Talk About It

Talk to each other about what sex means to your relationship. What do you want from sex? As the higher-drive person, talk about why sex is important to you. How does it make you feel when you don't have it? Don't assume that because one of you wants it less, it means less to them. Find out what would make the lower-drive person feel more open to sex. Avoid blame and judgment.

Think About the Problem Differently

Rather than taking it personally, think about your differing levels of sexual desire as you do about other differences in your personalities and preferences. You don't always like to eat the same things: You like to stay up late, she likes to go to bed early; she likes to watch *American Idol,* you don't. It may be that the person with less desire is simply programmed to have less of an interest in sex. It may not be tied to any deep psychological or relationship issues. And it doesn't necessarily mean the person loves you any less. It may be that that's just who they are. Thinking about libido as simply another aspect of each other's personality can help you be more objective about it.

Break the Advance/Rebuttal/Pout/ Resentment Cycle

Instead of feeling rejected and turning away from your partner to lick your emotional wounds when your sexual advance is turned down, acknowledge that your partner is not on the same page as you are. Ask if there's something else you can do for them, like give them a back rub or make them tea. Instead of feeling resentful that they don't want to have sex and sulking about it, stay open and connected. This will leave you both feeling more generous toward each other.

Let the Lower-desire Partner Come to You

Feeling subtle pressure to have sex can turn the lower-desire partner off even more. Yes, I realize the old "nudge, nudge, wink, wink" may seem like a playful, low-pressure way to communicate that you'd like to get intimate, but it's not going to work if the other partner isn't feeling it. They have to feel as if sex is genuinely off the table. This will allow them some breathing room to get there in their own time and on their own terms. This means that you don't push at the first sign of interest they show.

Go with the Flow

Realize that libidos naturally wane and shift depending on what's going on in our lives or what day of the week it is. Things like pregnancy, aging and illness also affect libido. Your current difference may be temporary. Just as you aren't always feeling madly in love with each other, you won't always feel sexually in sync. You've heard that old adage: The key to a successful marriage is that the two of you never fall out of love with each other at the same time. Your sexual incompatibility may just be temporary.

Stay Intimate in Other Ways

When sex isn't happening as often as one of you would like, an unexpected "I love you" on the way to the bathroom or a sexy neck nuzzle while he's doing the dishes at least keeps you physically in touch. Doing nice things for each other also helps. In fact, when you're both stressed and tired, doing the dishes can be pretty damn hot. Not exactly *Penthouse Forum* hot, I know, but those letters are made up anyway.

FEMALE ORGASM, OR WHY CAN'T I COME TOO?

Many women complain that they simply can't reach the Big O. And I'm not talking Oprah. Check out any supermarket magazine rack if you need further proof: "Easy Orgasms: How to Make Them Mind-Blowing and a Lot Less Work," "His & Hers Orgasms: How to Slow Him Down and Speed You Up." If you're having trouble achieving orgasm, here are some things to try:

On Second Thought, Stop Trying

Ironically, being aware of and thus self-conscious about whether or not you're going to get there is one of the biggest barriers to experiencing orgasm. Instead of enjoying the ride, you're lying there gritting your teeth, trying desperately to make it happen. Breathe, relax and stop trying so hard.

Practise Achieving Orgasm through Masturbation

If you haven't figured it out solo, it's going to be harder to let him know what gets you off. There is more specific guidance on how to practise in "Masturbation for Her" earlier in this book. If you've never used a vibrator, try one.

Don't Focus on Him Doing It "Right"

Even if you know exactly what gets you off through masturbation, it doesn't mean he has to do exactly the same thing. Try not to focus on whether he's doing it right or figuring it out. If he isn't, you can always get in there and help. In the meantime, enjoy the new pleasures he's bringing to the table, the ones you can't give yourself on your own. You might discover something new that gets you off.

Quiet the Voices in Your Head

This is not the time to be thinking of the grocery list. Focus instead on your body and how it feels. If you notice your mind wandering, bring it back into the moment. How are your toes feeling? Focus on the energy flowing between his body and yours.

Learn to Receive

Even with the gender equality we've achieved as a society, many women still spend way too much energy pleasing others, often at the expense of their own needs. Especially in the bedroom. For some reason, we get uncomfortable with all that attention, so we switch our focus to him. Kick back and really enjoy yourself, guilt-free. Trust me, there's nothing he'll like more than to see his work appreciated.

Be a Little Selfish

Imagine him saying, "Oh, it's okay, I don't really need to have an orgasm." I know, I know—sometimes you really don't need to. But let's face it, given the choice . . . Ditch the guilt.

Get a Head Start

If you know you're probably going to have sex later, cop a feel here and there throughout the day. (Be subtle: People may wonder why you're sitting at your desk with your hand down your pants.) Stimulate your mind. Fantasize about the things you'd like him to do to you. Anything to get your motor running.

Play with Yourself

Don't be afraid to play with yourself even when you're with him. Chances are, he'll love watching you touch yourself. If you're worried about making him feel inadequate, let him help. No need to bark orders—just gently guide his hand.

Get Past Your "I Must Come by Man, Not Machine" Barrier

Bringing in backup doesn't make your orgasm less legitimate. Use a vibrator or your fingers for extra clitoral stimulation.

Sometimes It's Just Not Going to Happen

It's okay to tell him it's just not happening for you. That way, you can shift the focus back to having fun. Stop worrying about how it's going to affect his ego. If he comes first, so what? And if he does come first and you still want to have an orgasm, ask if he'll go down on you. Or ask him to just hold you and play with your breasts, or penetrate you with his fingers or a toy, while you masturbate yourself to orgasm.

MALE ORGASM

WHY IS THIS TAKING SO LONG?

I definitely get more letters from women who can't come with a partner than I do from guys. Still, I get plenty of letters from guys who have a hard time coming. It's even tougher on men in some ways, because you're expected to orgasm pretty much as easily as you breathe. Like many of the women who write me, lots of guys say they can masturbate to orgasm but can't come during sex with her. Which makes sense. You know your own body and

when to change the rhythm, pressure, etc. without having to utter a word. It can be hard to communicate the idiosyncrasies of your own stick-handling practices. Given that you guys are generally less vocal than women, it's probably even harder for you to speak up about it. If this is an issue for you, here's some advice:

Give Her Some Hands-on Guidance

Place your hand over hers to gently direct her speed or pressure, or to guide her to where you'd like to be touched. Or masturbate in front of her to show her what works for you.

Switch Off the "It's Only Real Sex if I Come Inside Her" Voice in Your Head

Sure, intercourse is definitely designed to the advantage of the male orgasm, but that doesn't mean you're always going to come that way. There are lots of other ways to reach orgasm with a partner. You may be able to come more easily through oral or manual stimulation. Or, if you're comfortable, you can get her off and then masturbate yourself to orgasm while she fondles your boys or kisses your nipples.

Alleviate the Performance Pressure

If it feels like it's just not happening, remove the focus from orgasm altogether for a while. As with her, the more pressure you feel to have an orgasm, the less likely it's going to happen.

Rule Out Other Causes

Factors such as the heavy use of alcohol or recreational and/or prescription drugs (like tranquilizers and antidepressants) may also inhibit orgasm. Are you using condoms? If so, try thinner ones, or if you're in a monogamous relationship and STIs aren't an issue, consider an alternative birth control method. If you've ruled out physical causes (if you can achieve orgasm through masturbation, the problem isn't physical), more serious psychological issues may be at play, such as a fear of ejaculating inside a woman, impregnating her or transmitting a sexual disease to her. In this case, you had best seek professional counselling.

PREMATURE EJACULATION

The very terms "premature ejaculation" and "coming too soon" imply that there is some ideal amount of time to last. Or that you have to last in order for it to qualify as good sex. Most women (estimates put it at about 70 percent) don't orgasm through penetration alone. I hate to speak on behalf of your honey, but I suspect she'd be just as happy—if not more so—with lots of manual and oral stimulation and other kinds of sextracurricular activity mixed in with brief but enthusiastic intercourse as she would

be with a lengthy session of penetration-only sex.

However, if you want to learn to last longer, try these tips:

Practise the Stop/Start Method

While masturbating, take yourself to the edge of orgasm. Then stop, let the feeling subside and take yourself back to the brink again. Repeat this as often as you can until you become more aware of when you are reaching your point of no return and can stop before getting there. During sex, when you feel yourself getting close to orgasm, stop (squeezing your penis just below the head can help stop you going over the brink) and start again. Repeat to build up endurance.

Squeeze . . . and Squeeze . . .

Exercising your pelvic or PC muscles can improve ejaculatory control. Squeeze your pelvic muscles: Next time you're having a pee, stop yourself midstream. You just squeezed your PC muscles. Squeeze these several times whenever it occurs to you— while you're watching TV, while you're waiting for the kettle to boil—and you'll strengthen these muscles.

Don't Go Numb

Don't fall for any of those numbing creams they advertise to help control ejaculation.

These will only decrease sensation by numbing your penis (the numbing ingredient in most of these products is benzocaine, the same stuff you rub on the gums of teething babies), which is counterproductive. The key to not coming too quickly is to be more aware of the sensation in your penis and then learn how to control it.

ERECTILE DYSFUNCTION

It's perfectly normal for your penis to occasionally not cooperate. It may seem like it sometimes, but it's not a machine with an on/off switch. Fatigue, stress and too much booze are among the things that can put a wilt in your willy. So can worrying about maintaining your erection. If you lose it once, sheer nervousness about losing it again can be the very thing that makes you go limp. Sadly, we've come to rate a guy's entire sexual performance on the strength of his erection.

But erectile dysfunction—that is, not being able to get an erection—happens to lots of guys. An estimated twenty to thirty million men in North America, or about one in eight, can't get it up. And these aren't just older men, as most people think. While 25 percent of men experience some erectile dysfunction by age seventy-five, at least 8 percent of young adult men experience it from time to time.

An estimated 90 percent of erectile dys-

function cases are due to physical causes. Smoking and poor diet, for example, can eventually lead to hardened arteries that can't pump blood to the penis as efficiently. In some cases, causes that are not lifestyle-related, like diabetes or scar tissue on the penis, can lead to erectile problems. If the problem is purely physical, treatments such as injections, penile implants and, of course, erectile dysfunction drugs may be just the thing to get you standing at attention.

If you can still get an erection while sleeping or masturbating, or unexpectedly while standing in line at the supermarket, the plumbing clearly still works, so the problem might be psychological. If this is the case, a temporary pharmaceutical treatment might boost your confidence and get you back in the saddle. If the psychological problems run deeper, professional therapy may be necessary.

SAFER SEX

This book is aimed primarily at monogamous, heterosexual couples who might assume that condoms, sexually transmitted infections and safer sex aren't an issue. And to a certain extent you may be right. As long as you have both been tested for sexually transmitted infections and you are truly monogamous, you probably don't have a lot to worry about and you can lose the condoms (unless of course you're using them for contraception).

However, even if you think you're infection-free, know that certain sexually transmitted viruses, such as the human papillomavirus (HPV) and herpes, can be carried in your system even if you have no visible symptoms. This means they can be transmitted to your partner. And certainly, if you are involving outside partners in your sex life as a couple—like having a three-some—you need to protect yourselves.

Ultimately, if you have any concerns about the communication of STIs between you and your partner, you must use a condom during any type of penetrative sex.

These days, condoms come ribbed, textured, ultra thin, extra large, low odour, specially designed for her pleasure—the list goes on. So there's no excuse not to find a condom that works for you both. What? Your partner's a vegan? Just pick up some animal-product-free vegan condoms at your friendly neighbourhood sex shop. Heck, why not pick up a Swarovski-crystal-embossed case to carry them in while you're at it?

No matter what kind of condom you prefer, the important thing is that you make sure it is used and it is worn right. Here's a refresher course, just in case:

Check the expiry date. If it's been in your wallet for three years, ditch it. If the condom is brittle, stiff or sticky, discard it and use another.

If you're not circumcised, pull back your foreskin before putting on the condom. A drop or two of water-based lubricant (oil will destroy the latex) or saliva inside the tip of the condom will reduce any friction. Place the rolled-up condom over the tip of your penis, pinching the tip to leave space for your, er, deposit. Roll down the rim to win—I mean, all the way to the base of your penis. Take an occasional peek during sex to make sure the condom's still on and hasn't broken.

Be sure to wrap your hand around the base of the condom as you pull out so it doesn't slip off. Remove, tie a knot in it (to prevent spillage) and discard (in the garbage, not in the toilet or behind the door for Fido to find later).

Acknowledgements

Thanks first to the ever patient, practical and always inspirational Kate Cassaday, my editor at HarperCollins and the reason this book made its way into the world. I have to give special thanks to my superb emergency editrix and saviour Jane Warren, who helped dig me out when I wrote myself into a particularly tight corner. And big heaps of thanks to production editor Kelly Hope and to Sarah Wight for her meticulous copy-editing work. Thanks also to my literary agent, Anne McDermid, and the team at Anne McDermid and Associates, with a special thanks to Chris Bucci for all his help. Thanks to the team at the National Speakers Bureau, who always have my back. And thanks to our super models and to Deb G. for bringing them to us. To my dear friends and respected colleagues Kathy Buckworth, Karen LaRocca, Nicola Luksic and Tina Pittaway, I thank you dearly for your professional feedback and personal support. To the rest of my nearest and dearest, Li, Darcelle, Isabel, Sarah, Ilana, Char, Audrey, Wanda, Linda, Chuck, Thom, Jenny, Tara, Vanessa, Karen S. and the Fediuk clan, thanks for the love, the cheerleading and the superb listening skills.

To those who continue to work hard to make us all more sex-positive and who have inspired me in the almost two decades I've been writing about sex, thank you. Here in Canada, the folks at Come As You Are, Good for Her, Venus Envy, and Womyn's Ware, Cory Silverberg, Carlyle Jansen, Trina Read and Morpheus. In the United States, Candida Royalle, Tristan Taormino, Susie Bright, Midori and Dr. Marty Klein.

Thank you, Daniel, for your patience, kindness, true love, amazing talent and the stunning photographs in this book. And finally, as always, thanks to my ever insanely (I said insanely, not insane!) loving and supportive family. To all my siblings—too many to mention—I'd need to write another whole book to share all that you mean to me. To my dearly beloved father, still strong in our hearts and so much a part of who I am. And especially to my amazing eighty-eight-year-old mom. You inspire me every day.